Natural Bir

A clear, sensible explanation of this very effective method of
family planning, which attunes you to the cycles of your
own body in planning or preventing conception.

Natural Birth Control

A Guide to Contraception through Fertility Awareness

Katia & Jonathan Drake

Foreword by Dr Andrew Stanway

THORSONS PUBLISHING GROUP

Wellingborough, Northamptonshire

First published 1984
Second Edition 1987

British Library Cataloguing in Publication Data

Drake, Katia
Natural birth control.
1. Natural family planning
I. Title   II. Drake, Jonathan
613.9′434   RG136.5

ISBN 0-7225-0878-6

*Published by Thorsons Publishers Limited, Denington Estate,
Wellingborough, Northamptonshire, NN8 2RQ, England*

Printed in Great Britain by Woolnough Bookbinding,
Irthlingborough, Northants

1   3   5   7   9   10   8   6   4   2

Contents

Acknowledgements

This book has drawn extensively from the work of many researchers and clinicians who laid the scientific foundations.

In particular we wish to thank Dr Evelyn Billings for stimulating our interest, and Dr Anna Flynn and all at the NFP Centre, Birmingham, for setting us on the teaching road. Jean Johnson (National Promoter of NFP for the Catholic Marriage Advisory Council) kindly agreed to check the manuscript and always dealt with our numerous questions in a warm, encouraging and helpful way. The comments of Ilana Machover and Dr Yehudi Gordon helped greatly to clarify the text. Dr Mark Agius alerted us to the importance of Roetzer's work, and Georgie Vargas highlighted for us many of the political aspects of fertility awareness. Finally, we are grateful to all the women from whom we have learnt, and continue to learn, how to teach fertility awareness. The opinions expressed, though, are our own.

Foreword

With increasing evidence that there are side effects to many, if not all, of the existing methods of contraception used by most women during their fertile years, increasing numbers of people are seeking new methods that have no health risks. This book helps them do this.

'Natural Birth Control' is, of course, nothing new. Women have used an intimate knowledge of their fertility cycles to plan their families for centuries but today science has validated many of the old wives' tales that surround the subject and has at last made it acceptable rather than cranky.

Katia and Jonathan Drake have, with this book, filled a gap in the market. There have been several books on the subject already but most have their shortcomings and they are often too complicated and a bigger read than most people want or need.

In this little book, which can be read in an evening, all the salient information is clearly and honestly presented by a husband and wife team who teach fertility awareness and its use to women and other couples.

This kind of family planning or contraception is unlikely to do all the other methods out of business if only because it requires considerable motivation and care to make it work but for those who have religious prohibitions or medical problems with other methods this 'natural' way could be the answer they are looking for. Unfortunately, the whole subject has a bad name because most people (including many doctors) still think that natural birth control is the same as the rhythm method which so disastrously fails millions of Catholic couples. This is not the case. The sort of birth control that this book describes goes way beyond this primitive and unreliable method and as a result is much more effective as a contraceptive.

However good this contraceptive method is though and however well it is applied it will never be the answer to those couples who want to be free to have intercourse throughout the month in an unrestricted way. Natural family planning relies on other methods being used during the most fertile time which means that such a couple's contraceptive safety then depends on the alternative (usually barrier) method that they use. Given that barrier methods, properly used together with a spermicide, are very nearly as safe as the pill in contraceptive terms, this should not prove to be a problem for most couples, especially if they are planning a family as opposed to using a true contraceptive (which by definition ensures absolute safety from pregnancy).

With the increasing interest in more natural approaches to health generally, this book is likely to hit just the right note in those who want to have greater control over their bodies and their reproductive functioning. It is a book for the responsible woman who wants to know and understand more about herself and as such I can highly recommend it.

DR ANDREW STANWAY
M.B., M.R.C.P.

Preface —
A Personal Note

We began using natural birth control because we had to find an alternative to the usual methods of contraception. On the Pill Katia became very restless and disturbed without knowing why, her legs swelled and became hard, and she put on weight. A bad pelvic infection followed the fitting of a coil. It took over eighteen months for this condition to clear up, aided by careful nutrition and holistic medicine.

We wondered if it would be possible to have a family, but when we felt it was the right time to start trying, Katia got pregnant straight away! We knew when conception occurred, so it was amusing to be told by the hospital that our dates were correct: we assured them their ultra-sound scan was accurate! Our son was born 'on time' with no intervention whatsoever — a natural active birth — and we were all home three hours later.

Immediately after the birth our doctor asked us what method of contraception we were going to use. 'Natural birth control, of course!' we said. We were amazed to find how little many gynaecologists know about the signs of fertility which women can reliably observe themselves. Indeed, it is not uncommon for a young woman worried about a mid-cycle vaginal discharge to be reassured that there is no infection, and yet not to have its significance pointed out.

At 'family planning' clinics, which cater for the blanket demand for effortless contraception, you are unlikely to be advised on natural methods. If you are, it is only to be warned not to trust them! This advice is not based on a full understanding of the evidence. Women of all backgrounds have demonstrated that fertility awareness can readily be learnt, and that modern methods are highly effective at identifying the fertile times. However, dependence on something outside of yourself is usually seen to be more reliable! By being willing, though, to learn to observe your body's signals, you will soon discover that nature has given you a clear indication of your state of fertility.

We did not find a teacher when we wanted to learn natural birth control, so we decided to teach ourselves. Mary Shivandan's book *Natural Sex* (Hamlyn, 1979) gave us a good general perspective on NFP, but it is not a practical guide. Reading more widely, there always seemed to be an excessive amount of information on anatomy and physiology to wade through, and sometimes the tendency to moralize could be off-putting. Surely fertility awareness is for everyone to learn about!

The more we became interested and involved in natural birth control, the more we discovered that most people know very little about it. It was because of this that we felt we wanted to teach. So when Jonathan embarked on a course to become a qualified teacher of NFP, he was building on aspects of his earlier studies at medical school. This cleared up many of our questions, and we began to better understand why there are a number of different approaches to NFP. He had graduated in medicine in 1976, disillusioned with conventional medical approaches to most of the problems people present to their family doctors. Since then, he has been involved with alternatives, including the Alexander Technique and health education.

We will try, in this book, to give an up-to-date account of mainstream thinking in NFP and to explain the reasons for certain guidelines, so that you really know what you are doing. At the same time, we only include the most relevant medical information in the main body of the book (see the appendices for further information).

No book is, of course, a substitute for personal guidance. While this book can be used on its own, you will probably save yourself some initial uncertainty if you seek the help of a competent user or teacher of NFP (see 'Useful Addresses', page 93).

Many women find it fascinating learning to observe and live in tune with their fertility. We hope you find this an enjoyable and valuable experience as well.

KATIA AND JONATHAN DRAKE

Introduction

The aim of this book is to explain in clear and simple terms, the signs of fertility which any woman can observe within herself.

A man's fertility shows no cyclical variation, but in the course of the female cycle there are comparatively few days when it is possible to conceive. This fact is not taken into account by contraception applied in an all-or-nothing way, or by methods which suppress these natural variations in fertility.

The signs of fertility should be known by everyone on reaching sexual maturity or even earlier: it is knowledge for life, whether you are involved in a relationship or not. To realize that marked changes in mood and sensitivity may be linked with cyclical differences in hormones can be enormously liberating. Fertility awareness is a valuable monitor of normal healthy functioning, and it may enable certain problems to be detected at an early stage. With this knowledge, if you then decide to go on the Pill or have the IUD ('coil') fitted, at least you know what you will be interfering with! As well as being valuable in itself, fertility awareness can be used to avoid or achieve pregnancy — a true method of family planning.

Modern methods of natural birth control can be, if applied correctly, as effective as other means of contraception. The 'rhythm' method ('Vatican roulette'!) is a thing of the past. Changes in cervical mucus, body temperature and the cervix now give a reliable indication of your state of fertility, whether your cycles are long, short or irregular.

People are becoming increasingly wary about the hazards of the Pill and IUD, and are perhaps turning reluctantly to 'barrier' methods such as the diaphragm or condom. If so, why not be sure to use them just when they are really needed, at the most fertile time of the cycle?

Some couples experience difficulty in having a child. By observing and charting your cycles, you can find out if you are releasing an egg cell regularly, and thus identify what may be infrequent and brief fertile phases. The value of fertility awareness in preparing for pregnancy is that you will know when you conceived and therefore have a good idea of when your baby is due, so there will be less risk of an unnecessary induction of labour.

Fertility awareness is knowledge to be shared with your partner, and the mutual understanding it encourages can make an important contribution to your relationship. Together you become more responsible for an important area of your lives and less dependant on doctors.

At one time people only used natural family planning (NFP*) for traditional religious reasons. Today, as more of us question our relationship to each other and our environment, the need to live consciously in harmony with our fertility will be increasingly realized and welcomed.

* We use the term NFP to refer in general to fertility awareness and its applications; the term 'natural birth control' is used to emphasize the avoidance of pregnancy. 'Natural' is used, with some reservation, because of conventional usage by others in family planning, to signify the avoidance of side-effects associated with other, 'artificial', methods, and because we rely on what is given us to observe.

1.

The Fertility Cycle

Menstruation is such an obvious event, it is not surprising that the more subtle signs of fertility can easily be missed. Let's take an overview of these changes in the *fertility cycle*.

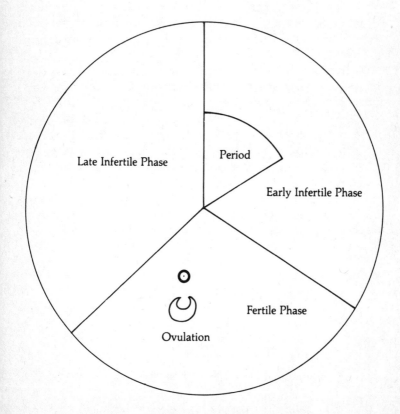

Figure 1. The phases of the fertility cycle.

By learning how to observe these changes and interpret their significance, you will come to appreciate how beautifully orderly your cycles actually are — even when they vary in length — and you will soon get to know exactly where you are at any point in your cycle. The fertility cycle can be divided up into three parts: the fertile phase around ovulation (the release of the egg cell or ovum from the ovary); and infertile phases before and afterwards (see Figure 1).

The facts of ovulation
Firstly, when does ovulation occur in the course of the cycle? There are myths about its timing: that it occurs two weeks after the period; that it can happen without warning at any time. In fact, it was established by scientific observation more than fifty years ago that ovulation takes place approximately two weeks *before* the following period. And once it has happened, there will not be another ovulation in that cycle, unless within twenty-four hours of the first. (This unusual event could be the cause of non-identical twins.)

So, irrespective of cycle-length, it is the number of days before ovulation that varies: the phase after ovulation tends to stay constant, within a normal range of 12 to 16 days.* Let's look at how this works in the following example (see Figure 2). By convention, the days of the cycle are counted from the first day of the period to the day before the next one, and so, in a 25-day cycle, ovulation is likely to occur between days 10-14, and with a 35-day cycle, between days 20-24.

The next question is, how long does the egg live for? It is now thought that it lasts no longer than six to twelve hours, but an outside limit of twenty-four hours is usually allowed for.

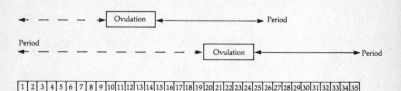

Figure 2.   The constant phase after ovulation.

* Exceptionally, with very short cycles, ovulation may occur as little as 10 days before menstruation.

Sperm survival

The other main factor determining the fertile phase is the timing of intercourse in relation to ovulation. During the infertile phases of the cycle, sperm perish within a few hours in the acidic conditions in the vagina. Near ovulation, a particular type of mucus is produced which can keep the sperm alive for three days or even, very exceptionally, up to five days.

Thus, the combined fertility of a couple *should* be no more than three to five days. In practice, modern methods of fertility awareness allow you to identify ovulation to within two days either side, and so the length of the fertile phase is likely to be about a week to ten days.

The rhythm method

This knowledge about the timing of ovulation and the life-span of the egg and sperm was used to work out the formulae on which the rhythm or calendar method is based. From the shortest and longest of a number of recent cycles (at least six to twelve), it is possible to calculate the *probable* time of the fertile phase. However, each new cycle is an unknown quantity, and the only value of the rhythm method on its own is in spacing or delaying pregnancies. It cannot cope with irregularities in cycle length. Complicating factors such as stress, illness or travel can delay or block ovulation and the cycle will then be much longer than usual: there is no such thing as a 'missed' period. So, many pregnancies occurred because cycles were unexpectedly prolonged by external conditions. The other reason for the failure of the rhythm method is that the calculated fertile phase covers two weeks or more. Such a long time of abstinence is neither popular or easy for most couples!

What was required, then, was clear accurate indication of the fertile phase whatever the particular circumstances of the cycle.

Minor indicators

Some women seem to know intuitively whether they are fertile from a number of possible physical and psychological changes occurring around mid-cycle:

- A short-lived sharp stabbing pain, or a dull ache on one side of the lower abdomen lasting a day or so. The cause is now thought to be the stretching of the ovarian capsule.
- Increased retention of fluid may cause generalized effects, or the breasts may become sore and tender, or there may

be abdominal bloating, or a feeling of fullness and pressure in the genitals.

- A pink or brown discharge or spotting of blood, or even actual bleeding — an effect of high oestrogen levels on the lining of the womb.
- A change in sensitivity. There may be an increase in energy or sexual desire, or a feeling of irritability or tiredness.
- Changes in the oiliness of the hair and skin and the clarity of the complexion.

Do these signs reliably identify the fertile time? In practice they vary from cycle to cycle, or they may not be experienced at all. Furthermore, they do not clearly mark the beginning and ending of fertility, which is of more practical value to us than knowing precisely when ovulation occurs. It is good to appreciate their significance and to relate them to the main signs of fertility, *but they cannot be depended upon*.

Major signs

The first step towards solving the problem of defining the limits of fertility was the temperature method, which was introduced in about 1960. It involves taking your temperature on waking up in the morning. At, or immediately following, ovulation there is a small but distinct rise in temperature. Once three consecutive higher temperatures have been recorded, you are in the late infertile phase of the cycle.

The big disadvantage of this method is that it does not give warning of ovulation. You can only have unprotected intercourse in the late part of the cycle, and if cycles are long the waiting can be arduous! And so the temperature method is only a partial answer. Can anything give sufficient warning of ovulation?

If women are asked this question, some wonder about the significance of the vaginal discharge which feels as though a period is coming, but which occurs around the middle of the cycle. The earliest reference to this mucus 'symptom' (as if it were an illness) in the medical literature was in the 1850s. Over the next hundred years, as times changed and it became respectable and necessary, the bulk of research into fertility went into developing artificial methods of contraception — culminating in the Pill and the IUD. It is remarkable how little attention nature's signs received by comparison.

In the cervical mucus method (sometimes called the Billings

or Ovulation Method) changes in sensation and the appearance of mucus at the entrance to the vagina are noted. There is commonly a build-up of mucus over six days and then a decline as ovulation is finishing.

Changes in cervical mucus and temperature are the main indicators of fertility, and a simple daily check of the cervix itself can be added if you wish — since it is the source of the external mucus sign.

Generally it is best to use a combination of methods (variously called 'double-check', 'muco-thermic' or 'sympto-thermal'). This is for two reasons. The first is that, by gaining experience of all the methods, you can then select whichever method or combination of methods fits your particular circumstances. The second is that, while the cervical mucus and temperature methods can be 97-99 per cent effective, in practice you are more likely to come close to achieving this if you use a *combination* of methods (see Appendix A, page 80). It is only a little extra effort at first, and you will be surprised how easily fertility awareness becomes a part of your life, taking no more trouble than brushing your teeth!

Fertility awareness and adolescence

What better time to start learning fertility awareness than when periods start! It enables you to tune into yourself and understand some of the ups and downs of this time of rapid development.

On average, ten years pass before the reproductive system matures fully. Until then, it is more common for cycles to be anovulatory (that is, no egg is released). One in two of cycles are likely to be anovulatory in the first year, and that gradually lessens until only one in thirty are anovulatory. Also, the length of time between ovulation and the next period may be quite short. If there are less than nine days of elevated temperatures, the cycle is unlikely to be fertile. Your early charts will reflect these gradually changing and maturing patterns. Adolescence does not call for the Pill in order to 'regularize' your periods! Its effect at this time, by imposing an artificial rhythm on you, is to thwart the normal development of your reproductive system, and it may delay the settling-down of your cycles into their own natural, regular rhythm.

The following chapters explain how to observe and chart your fertility cycles. You can start with the temperature method or the cervical mucus test, or learn both at the same time.

2.

The Temperature Method

The temperature method transformed NFP. For the first time it was possible to make a reliable judgement about fertility, however long or short cycles were. From the chart you could see if ovulation had occurred and, if it had, the late absolutely infertile part of the cycle could be determined.

The temperature method of birth control can have 99 per cent effectiveness, approaching that of the Pill. It is a useful method to start with because, in the first complete cycle you chart, you will be able to have unprotected intercourse once you have identified the temperature shift. In the long-term, its value as a single method of fertility awareness is greatest for couples who have the strongest need to avoid pregnancy and are prepared to put up with long periods of abstinence; or for those willing to accept a slightly higher method failure rate, and who wish to make use of a barrier method until ovulation is over.

We taught an orthodox Jewish couple who were anxious to avoid a further pregnancy for medical reasons. The wife had been fitted with a coil. This device, which may work by setting up an irritation of the lining of the womb, prolonged her periods for 14 days out of — on average — 28-day cycles. The effect on their sex life was disastrous, because, according to Jewish Law, one must avoid any contact during menstruation and for seven clear days afterwards. Every cycle, then, they had to wait until day 22, by which time ovulation was well over. So what was the point of the coil? By substituting the temperature method for the coil, more days would be made available for intercourse, and the risk of anaemia, fertility-threatening infection and the possibility of ectopic pregnancy (outside the womb) from the coil, could be much reduced.

You may think that taking your temperature every day sounds

a lot of trouble — after all, you're not ill! Many women find it an easy routine, and that it is exciting to see the distinct changes associated with ovulation.

Temperature recording

The temperature is taken as soon as you wake up in the morning. This is known as 'basal body temperature'; that is, the body temperature at rest. It does not appear to make any significant difference whether you stay in bed or not, but if you forget to take your temperature for some minutes after getting up, activity will then have disturbed the accuracy of the recording.

The other main condition is to have had at least three hours' sleep and, if you've had to get up, to have been back in bed for an hour or more before you take your temperature. Even if your life-style is not regular, so long as you note any disturbances *at the time*, you should still find that you can interpret your charts fairly easily. Don't give up, then, if you forget to take your temperature one morning, or you think the recording is going to be all over the place.

It is often said you *must* take your temperature at the same time each morning. This is because it is known that body temperature shows a variation in the course of the day, being at its lowest in the early hours of the morning. Later on in the chapter we shall discuss how it is possible to make a correction for different waking times.

In order to obtain accurate readings easily, a special *fertility* glass mercury thermometer is recommended. It has a narrower range of temperatures than the usual clinical thermometer: 35°39°C (96°100°F), instead of 35°42°C (94°108°F). You can buy a fertility thermometer at a chemist or drug-store or from an NFP organization (and in Britain it can be obtained free on prescription — if your doctor is co-operative!)

It probably makes no difference to the reliability of the recording whether the temperature is taken by mouth, rectally or vaginally. The bulb of the fertility thermometer is bigger than the clinical thermometer and it takes longer for the mercury to rise. The thermometer should be left in the same place under the tongue in the closed mouth for at least five minutes (three minutes for the other routes), and nothing, of course, should be drunk just beforehand. Whichever method you decide on, stick to it throughout the cycle because rectal and vaginal temperatures are slightly higher than oral ones.

Plastic digital thermometers are now available which can serve as well as the traditional glass mercury thermometers. Their advantages are that they are virtually unbreakable and they give you a numerical read-out. Since they normally register in one minute though, it is advisable to wait for a couple of minutes with your mouth closed before inserting the thermometer, in order to get an accurate reading. Use either a Centigrade one reading to two decimal places, or a Fahrenheit one.

You can record your daily temperatures on the chart in the morning, or it may be more convenient for you to wait until the evening when you note any other observations made during the day. Unless the surrounding temperature is likely to be higher than your body temperature or the thermometer is left on a sunny window-sill, the mercury thermometer will not show a temperature altered from the morning. Before you go to sleep, make sure it has been shaken down and is ready by the bed for the next morning. (Shaking it over the bed may save a broken thermometer!) It is handy to keep a spare thermometer, so that you are not without at the critical time of the cycle when you want to be sure of accurately determining your temperature shift. If you have a spare, it is a good idea to take your temperature with one thermometer after the other one morning so that you can calibrate your spare one: they may vary by 0.1°C (0.2°F), which could be critical.

There are a number of different charts you can use to record your observations. Some women use graph-paper, but it is easier to use special charts. You can make photocopies of the chart on page 89 of this book, or ask one of the NFP teaching organizations to send you copies. The temperature is marked by a dot in the centre of the square and, if in doubt about which reading to take, the general rule to follow is to round *down* to the nearest reading. Most charts allow you to record your temperature accurate to 0.05°C (0.1°F).

The temperature shift
In Figure 3, you will see an example of a typical temperature record. There is an obvious rise in temperature on day 16, and it stays up until just before the next period, when it begins to fall. This pattern of lower and then higher temperatures is called a *biphasic* recording.

The temperature rise takes place at or after ovulation. It is caused by the ovarian hormone *progesterone*, which also inhibits the release of further eggs, except within one day of the first. You must wait for three consecutive higher temperatures to be sure that this process is over and that you are infertile for the rest of the cycle. *On the first two days of higher temperatures you may still be fertile.*

Many charts are easy to interpret at a glance. There are simple criteria you can use to determine the temperature shift when it is not quite so obvious. The easiest rule to apply is as follows: *A temperature shift has taken place once there are three daily consecutive undisturbed temperatures, all of which are higher than the previous six lower temperatures. The rise in temperature is at least 0.2°C (0.4°F) and takes place between the last lower and one of the three higher temperatures.* Commonly this rise occurs abruptly from one day to the next, but sometimes it is gradual or in steps over a number of days (see Figure 4).

Sometimes, for no apparent reason, there may be a spiky temperature in the previous six which is usually 0.2°C (0.4°F) or more higher than the temperatures on either side. *One* such temperature can safely be ignored, whether you know the reason for it or not. Nor do you need to include the first four temperatures of the cycle; the temperature may still be falling from the previous cycle (see Figure 5).

So, on the chart, from day 5 onwards, you count out six temperatures to see if the next one is at a higher level. If no rise has taken place, then day by day the six temperatures are re-counted so that, when the rise takes place, it occurs in relation to the six temperatures immediately before. It can be very helpful to draw a 'cover-line': that is, a line immediately above the highest of the lower temperatures, to be sure that all three subsequent temperatures are at a higher level.

What are the reasons for this 'three-over-six' rule? Firstly, let's look at the probable time of ovulation in relation to the temperature graph.

Estimating ovulation
Research using hormone measurements shows that ovulation can occur as early as the fifth lower temperature, and as late as the second higher temperature (including a second ovulation). It is most likely to happen around the previous three lower temperatures (see Figure 6). It used to be believed that the lowest point of the graph denoted the day of ovulation, but it has now been shown to be more variable than that.

For our purposes, trying to pin-point the day of ovulation is

Figure 3. A typical temperature record.

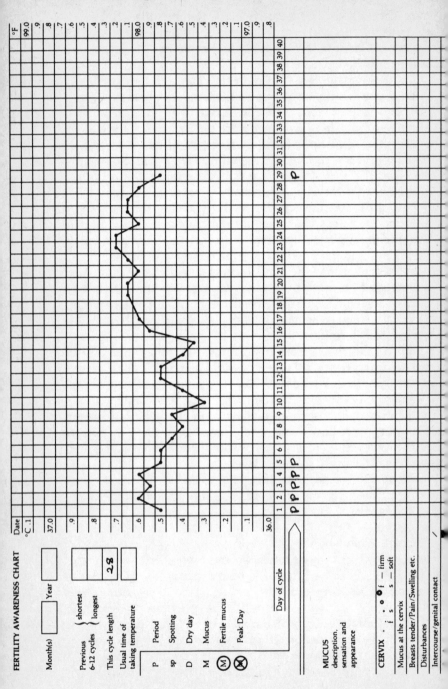

Figure 4.   The 'three-over-six' rule.

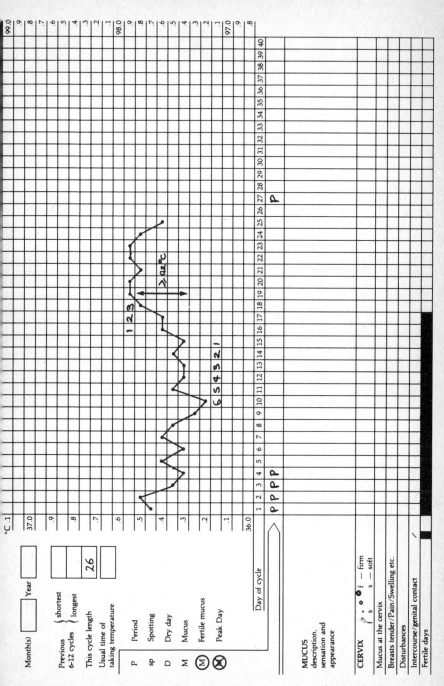

Figure 5.   Ignoring certain temperatures.

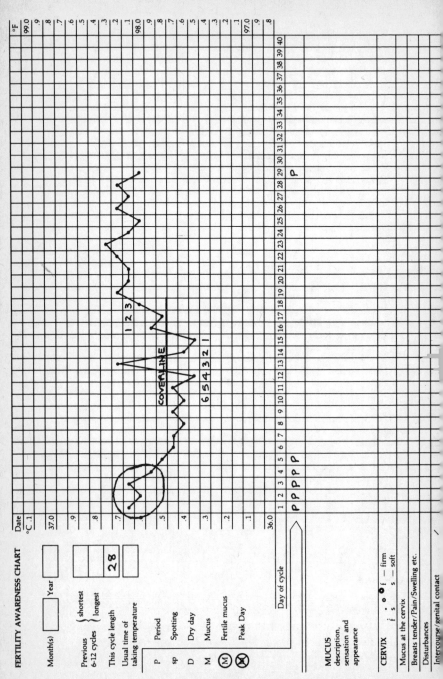

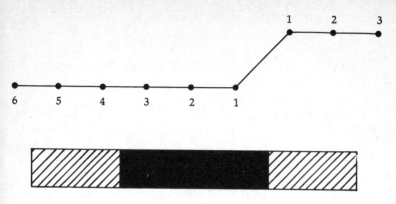

Figure 6.   Ovulation in relation to the temperature method.

not as important as identifying the limits of fertility. We cannot narrow down ovulation any more precisely than to two days either side of the most probable day. Even the most sophisticated hormone tests cannot do much better!

The question is: why are *six* lower temperatures needed? The answer is an empirical one — that it works. In most cycles there are more than six temperatures before the shift, and some authorities recommend that all of them should be fitted underneath the cover-line (omitting the first four and any obvious spikes). This strict rule sometimes places the temperature shift rather late in the cycle, and for most purposes, the 'three-over-six' rule is highly reliable.

Temperature disturbances
There are a number of factors which can affect the basal body temperature. Such disturbances should be marked on the chart *at the time*. How do you deal with them in the interpretation of the temperature record?

Oversleeping. It is important to record *when* you take your temperature, if at a different time from the usual hour. This is especially likely to happen at weekends. The body temperature rises by approximately 0.1°C/0.2°F (it ranges from 0.05°C/0.1°F to 0.15°C/0.3°F) for each hour later that you take it between 5 and 11 a.m., and so a suitable correction should be made.

It would be useful, one morning when you are lying-in, to take your temperature at intervals to see how much it actually changes.

Some people find that the rise is very small and the regularity of temperature-taking such that it is not necessary to correct the temperature reading at all. Others find that it makes a big difference to the clarity of the chart. Until you find out how much your temperature changes, do not assume a bigger change than the lower limit of the range; that is, 0.05°C (0.1°F) per hour. Figure 7 shows how one woman, *knowing* that her temperature changed by 0.1°C per hour, circled those temperatures disturbed by a different time of waking, and only included the *adjusted* temperatures in the temperature curve. Only in this situation, when you know exactly what the adjustment factor is, can you include any number of time-adjusted temperatures in the previous six lower or following three higher temperatures.

Illness. If you are feeling unwell, you will soon see that there is a marked difference between the sharp rise in temperature due to sickness and the small sustained rise associated with ovulation (see Figure 8). Emotional upset, shock or excitement may also produce spiky temperatures. Remember that you can count only one of these disturbed temperatures amongst the previous lower six. If the disturbance occurs at the time of the temperature shift, you must wait until it has passed before counting the three higher temperatures.

Drugs. Alcohol nearly always causes a rise in temperature in moderate amounts, if not a hangover! Rarely it may depress body temperature, as can aspirin.

If you find you often take pain-killers or consciousness-altering drugs do you know why you depend on them? The body has its own intelligence, and by abusing it you destroy its sensitivity. Pain can be a way of drawing your attention to the fact that something is wrong. There are often multiple causes; diet, emotional reactions, mechanical and postural factors are among the first to look at, and they are within your power to change (see Further Reading, page 91).

Anovulatory cycles. In a small proportion of cycles, ovulation does not take place, and you will not see the typical biphasic graph. If the first cycle you record is like this, it can be a cause for concern, unless you are aware of the possibility (see Figure 9). Anovulatory cycles occur more frequently in the early or late reproductive years. The next period comes around the time you

Figure 7. Adjusting the temperature record according to waking time.

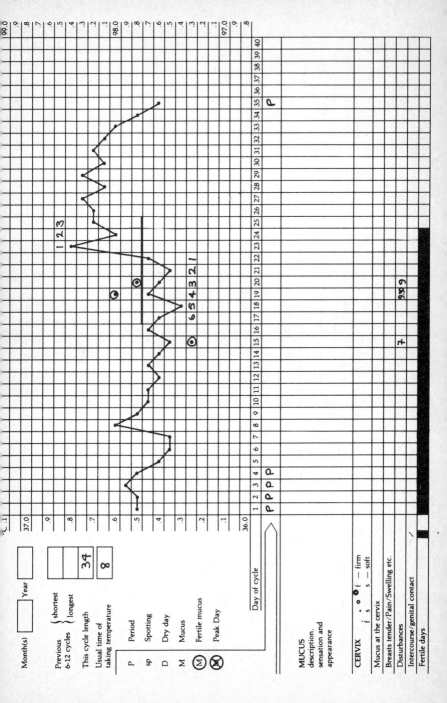

Figure 9.   An anovulatory cycle.

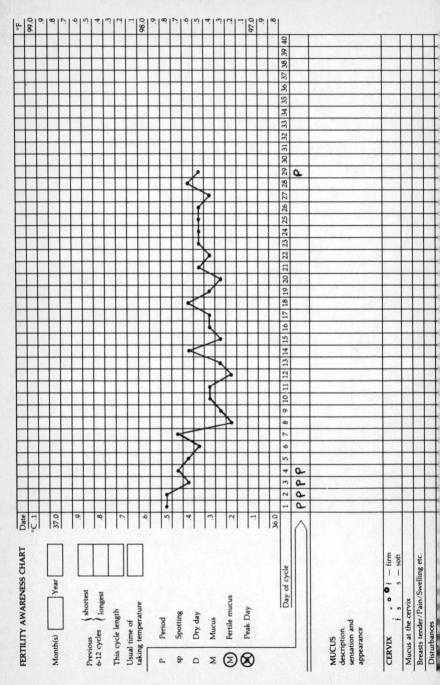

Figure 8. Fever and the temperature record.

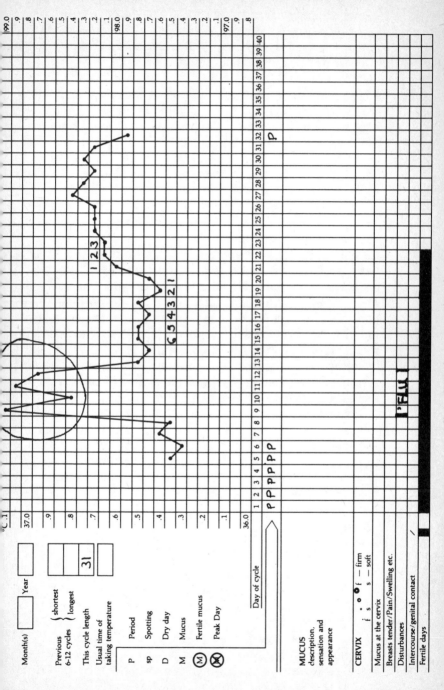

would normally expect it. From the temperature record alone, you cannot know which days in such a cycle are infertile. The mucus observation (see Chapter 3) and cervical changes will help you decide whether you are infertile or not.

Travel. Any circumstances which 're-set' the natural rhythms of the body are likely to make reliable temperature recording impossible for some time. Examples include crossing time-zones rapidly (air travel) and changing patterns of shift work. It may take the body some days — and perhaps a week or more — to adjust to such changes. Slower-paced travelling may delay or block ovulation, but the temperature record (and mucus and cervix changes) should accurately reflect your state of fertility.

Pregnancy. The temperature starts to drop just before menstruation begins. If it has stayed up for more than twenty days, pregnancy is highly likely. You may already *know* you are pregnant. It does give you, though, an objective indication of pregnancy before standard tests become positive. If the temperature stays up for longer than usual, and then a heavy painful period arrives with plenty of clots, it may mean an early miscarriage — nature's unfit conception.

Following a miscarriage or an abortion, depending on how advanced the pregnancy was, there is also likely to be some disturbance before cycles return to normal.

In circumstances when you have what seems to be an unduly long cycle, if the temperature has not risen it can be quite a relief to know that you have not ovulated and that you cannot possibly be pregnant. The danger with long cycles is assuming — without any evidence — that ovulation must be over. This is the surest recipe for an unplanned pregnancy.

Summary
The temperature method is a highly reliable way of determining ovulation and the late infertile phase of the cycle. It is especially useful while you are learning the other methods, because in the first cycle you chart, you should be able to have unprotected intercourse with confidence, once you have identified three higher temperatures.

The disadvantage of the temperature method alone is that it does not give you warning of ovulation and the start of the fertile phase. This is where the cervical mucus method (and cervix) come in.

3.

The Cervical Mucus Method

Not only does cervical mucus warn you of the imminence of ovulation, but it is a vital factor in the process of conception. Sperm die within a few hours in the normally acidic environment of the vagina. In ideal conditions, though, they may still be capable of fertilizing the egg for three days (or even, very unusually, up to five days).

Most women can readily identify their own mucus pattern. It requires no special tests or equipment and just a few seconds of observation at intervals during the course of the day.

The mucus is produced within the cervix — the lowermost part

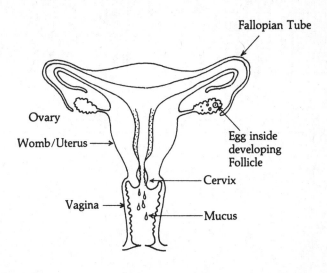

Figure 10. The female reproductive system.

Figure 11. Charting cervical mucus.

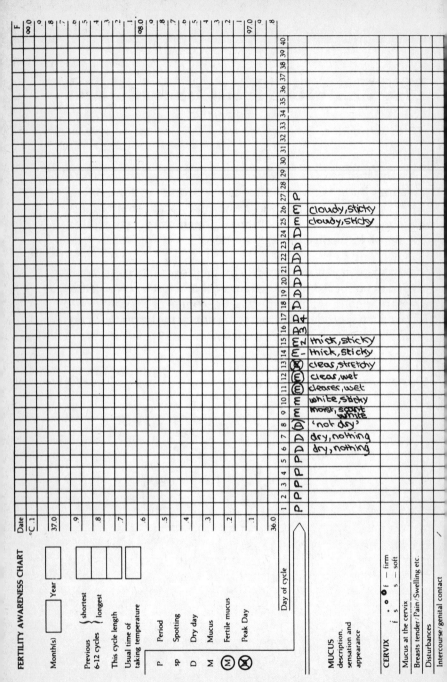

of the womb — and comes to the outside by the action of gravity (see Figure 10). There is no need to examine yourself internally with this method.

Probably the most convenient time for you to check for mucus is whenever you go to the toilet. You should ask the following questions. What is the sensation at the entrance to my vagina? Do I feel dry, or wet, or moist? Is there any mucus to be seen on the underwear or by wiping with tissue before and after urinating? What is its consistency, colour and elasticity? You will soon learn to distinguish between fertile-type mucus and less fertile mucus, or sometimes infertile mucus — depending on whether it occurs before or after ovulation.

Fertile mucus produces a wet, lubricative or slippery sensation at the entrance to the vagina. It is thin and watery, clear or slightly cloudy and, when gently stretched between the fingers it forms elastic threads. Occasionally, it may be pink or brown or spotted with blood.

Less fertile or infertile mucus is characteristically thick, opaque and sticky, and if you try to stretch it between the fingers a couple of times or so it breaks. Sometimes it is pasty or flaky and crumbly, so low is the water content.

Charting mucus

If you look at the chart shown in Figure 11 you will see that there is a space in which to enter the description of the mucus. It is important to note both the sensation you have experienced and the appearance of mucus — if any — in your own words. Unless you are clear about what you have observed, you will not know which kind of mucus is present. It will happen on some days that your mucus changes in quality in the course of the day, or you appear to have two kinds of mucus present at once, in which case when you come to record your observations at the end of the day, you should note the more fertile mucus.

There is a place on the chart just above the mucus description to record the kind of vaginal secretion you experience on each day. It is helpful to use a simple code so that you can see at a glance the pattern of mucus that is emerging. You can devise your own code, or you can follow the one used in this book (or the Billings colour scheme):

Period — P (red)
Spotting of blood — sp (red dots)

Dry days, no mucus — D (green)
Mucus, of less fertile type — M (yellow)
Fertile mucus — Ⓜ (white)

Now let's look in detail at some typical mucus patterns. It is important to bear in mind that no two patterns are exactly the same; your own patterns are unique to you and will vary to some extent from month to month. By understanding the principles behind the following charts, you should have a good idea of how to interpret your situation.

The classical pattern. When the period ends, there is a positive feeling of 'nothingness', of dryness. It may be itchy and slightly unpleasant, and there is no mucus to be seen at all.

Then the sensation of dryness changes. It may not be immediately replaced by one of wetness, but by dampness or stickiness, or you may notice a feeling of being no longer dry. This signifies that the hormone oestrogen is beginning to rise and ovulation is on its way. In the early infertile days, the cervix is sealed off by a thick plug of mucus. As it begins to ripen under

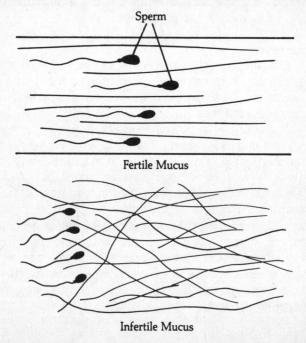

Sperm

Fertile Mucus

Infertile Mucus

Figure 12.　The penetrability of fertile and infertile mucus.

the influence of oestrogen, early mucus is produced and soon finds its way to the outside. When there is enough to observe, it will be seen to be the less fertile type. Its function is to make the vagina more alkaline and less hostile to sperm. In addition, it filters out immature and defective sperm so that only the most healthy are favoured.

As the oestrogen rises even higher, more mucus is produced and its water and salt content increases.* This is the more fertile-type mucus. If you look at it under a microscope, you can see many open channels which facilitate the transport of the sperm (see Figure 12). Sometimes this mucus is so profuse and stretchy it resembles the raw white of an egg.

Peak day is the last day of fertile mucus. It is called 'peak' because it is the day around which it is most likely that ovulation will take place. The time period for possible ovulation has been shown to be from two days before, to two days after peak day. Peak may not be the day of the greatest amount of fertile mucus, or the most stretchy; there may be only a residual feeling of wetness. It is identified retrospectively, that is, the following day there is a change back to the less fertile mucus or to dryness. Peak day is marked on the chart by Ⓧ

You will also notice that the days after peak have been numbered 1, 2, 3 and 4. This is because the first three days after peak are still potentially fertile, but from the evening of the fourth day past peak you are in the late infertile phase of the cycle. Why is this? If you remember, ovulation can happen up to two days after peak day. A further day must be added on to allow for the possibility of a second ovulation, and then a final day for the life-span of the egg. How is it possible for fertility to be maintained when fertile mucus is no longer present? One reason is that the less fertile mucus may still allow *some* sperm to get through. The other explanation is that there is some evidence that, included in their three-to-five day possible survival time, the sperm may be stored within the cervix for some time before travelling on to meet the egg.

So, in the chart shown in Figure 11, days 8 until the evening of day 17 are potentially fertile. Just before the period came, after a number of dry days, there were two days of mucus. This occasionally happens as the cervix opens slightly to allow menstruation to flow.

---

* It may have a 'glassy' appearance.

Figure 13. A continuous pattern of mucus.

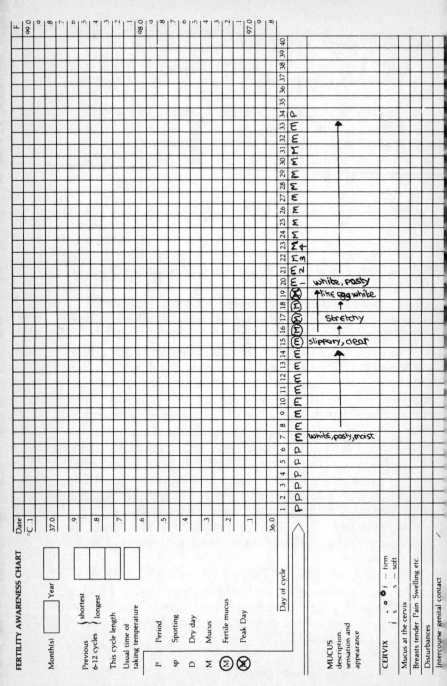

Figure 14.   The effect of stress in delaying ovulation.

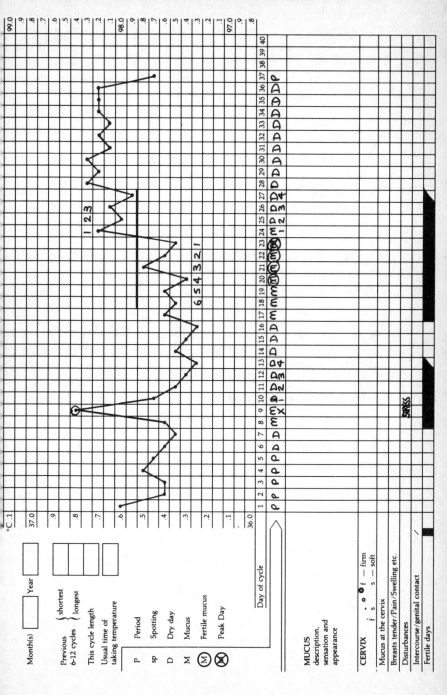

Continuous mucus. Some women have no days of dryness after the period ends, even in normal-length cycles. There always seems to be a small amount of 'mucus' present (see Figure 13). Its characteristic feature is that it stays the same from day to day, and in no way resembles fertile mucus. In order to distinguish between cervical mucus and vaginal cells, some women find the 'glass water test' useful. Drop some of the 'mucus' into a glass of water. If it is predominantly cervical mucus, it will stay separated from the water; if it dissolves, it is likely to be mainly made up of vaginal cells.

In the classical pattern described previously, the early mucus that appears has slightly fertile properties; the situation is that oestrogen is rising and ovulation is well on its way. When there is a pattern of continuous mucus, *any change* — in amount, or to a more fertile mucus — marks the ending of this basically infertile pattern and the beginning of the fertile phase. It is here that using an additional indicator, for example, checking the cervix, can be very helpful.

Scanty mucus. There may be so little mucus that it is virtually impossible to go by visual appearance and sensation then becomes very important. It does not take long to develop sensitivity; blind women have learnt to use the cervical mucus method successfully.

There is a simple procedure you can try (a *Kegel exercise*) to help you determine the sensation at the entrance to the vagina if you are not sure what it is. By contracting the muscles around the vagina (the same muscles are used if you try to stop urinating in mid-stream), and then relaxing, any discharge is helped down and the lips of the vaginal opening (the labia) move against each other. You should then be able to distinguish between true dryness; lessening of dryness; dampness, moistness or stickiness; and a wet, slippery or lubricative sensation.

Interpreting your cycles
With a little practice and application of the principles involved, an easy and natural feel for your fertility cycles should soon develop. In a small proportion of women, however, nothing resembling fertile mucus can be observed. In this case, you must learn to identify your own particular build-up of mucus, and peak day is the last day of this mucus before dryness returns. You may have noticed that the odour of your mucus varies at different times of the cycle. As mucus becomes more fertile, it has a sweeter

smell (and taste) compared with the sharper, more vinegary characteristics of the less fertile or infertile mucus.

If you find that no pattern at all emerges after a few cycles — and you have checked to be sure you know what you are looking for — your fertility may be low (see Chapter 9).

Mucus disruption
Now let's consider those factors which are likely to disturb the mucus sign.

Infection. An infected discharge — depending on the cause — will be irritating, smelly, profuse or yellow. Medical tests are necessary to identify the infective organism, and therefore determine an appropriate treatment.

In the meantime, if you think that it is probably a yeast infection ('thrush'), there is a simple home remedy worth trying. An imbalance in your general health can affect the acidity of the vagina so that the healthy, protective bacteria present in normal conditions are displaced. Early douching with 'live' yogurt (from a healthfood shop) helps restore healthy conditions, makes you feel more comfortable and may even cure the thrush.

An infected discharge will make it difficult to observe the subtle changes in mucus. It is a time to avoid intercourse altogether, because apart from delaying the healing process, there is bound to be a ping-pong effect where you and your partner pass the infection back and forth.

Drugs and hormonal disturbances. Drugs that affect mucus production include synthetic female hormones (see page 62) major tranquillizers and possibly anti-histamines and marijuana.

An under- or over-active thyroid gland may interfere with ovulation and the production of mucus.

Stress. This includes any challenge which demands adaptation to changing conditions. Common examples are illness, travel, fatigue, emotional upset and excitement. Dieting and excessive vigorous exercise may also have a profound effect on the hormone system via the brain centres. There are three possible consequences for fertility:

1. The disturbance has no apparent effect, and the mucus pattern develops as normal.

2. Ovulation is delayed until either the stress has passed or there has been a successful adaptation to it (see Figure 14). This is the apparent 'double peak' phenomenon. It is here that the temperature method is useful in indicating which patch of mucus coincided with ovulation. In extreme circumstances, ovulation and menstruation may be suppressed for many months or years (for example in anorexia nervosa, and in concentration camps).

3. Ovulation may not occur at all, yet the period comes around the usual time. There may be dryness throughout, or the mucus pattern may reflect the fluctuating hormone levels.

Summary

The beauty of the cervical mucus method is its basic simplicity and wide range of application. As a method of birth control, it has a potential effectiveness of at least 97 per cent, and it is the most efficient means of timing intercourse in order to achieve pregnancy.

The fertile phase begins as soon as there are any signs of a change from dryness. Otherwise, if there is a continuous pattern of mucus, it is essential to double-check the change to fertile mucus by another indicator. The beginning of the late infertile phase is from the evening of the fourth day past peak, which is the last day of fertile mucus.

4.

Checking the Cervix

Monitoring changes directly at the cervix gives you valuable information about your state of fertility. It is the cervix itself, affected by the relative amounts of oestrogen and progesterone, which produces the mucus you detect externally. Not only is it possible to feel the degree of 'ripeness' of the cervix, but you may be able to catch very early evidence of mucus before it comes down to the outside of the vagina.

The main value of the cervix as another indicator is that it can be used as a double check, with the cervical mucus method, for the beginning of the fertile phase. In circumstances where cycles are of variable length, and following childbirth or approaching the menopause, it can add confidence in interpreting the external mucus sign, especially if you have any difficulty in deciding what is happening externally.

Making friends with your cervix!
Some of us were brought up on the idea that it was quite wrong to touch *down there* at all, let alone fiddle around inside — that was the province of the doctor, armed with his speculum! There is sometimes the anxiety that you might damage yourself or cause an infection by interfering with yourself in this way. Such fears have no foundation, if you just observe simple precautions; be gentle with yourself, ensure that your nails are not too long and that your hands are moderately clean. (You wouldn't expect your partner to sterilize his penis!)

In certain women's self-help groups, you can learn to use a plastic speculum and mirror (obtainable from a chemist) to observe what is going on inside. The sense of touch, though, is extraordinarily acute, and with a little practice, you will be able to identify the changes at your cervix with no special equipment and the minimum of trouble. If you've used a diaphragm or felt for the threads of an IUD, you will already have a good idea of where to find your cervix. You will know when you've found it when you locate what feels like a smooth indented ball — quite different from the spongy texture of the vaginal wall.

Which posture you use to examine the cervix will also affect its position. Experiment until you have found a comfortable one in which you can most easily feel you cervix, and then use this position every time. You could try putting one leg up on a chair or side of the bath, or squatting. You can then feel for the cervix by inserting one or two fingers into the vagina. If necessary, the cervix can be made more accessible by gently bearing down, or using the other hand to press lightly down on the lower abdomen. Ensure that your bladder is empty because this will affect the position of the cervix.

Position. Early and late in the cycle, at the times of infertility, the cervix is low in position (see Figure 15). You may also notice it feels tilted in the vagina. In the fertile phase it rises gradually higher, perhaps by 2-3 cm (1 inch), straightening in position in the vagina. Once ovulation has occurred, it returns more quickly to a lower position. This is due to the effect of oestrogen on the supporting structures of the womb which retract slightly, and hence draw up the cervix.

If you begin looking for the cervix at the most fertile time, you may wonder why you can't find it, and whether you have one at all! In some women, the cervix may be especially high anyway and slightly to one side of the mid-line. If you start checking the cervix in the late infertile phase when it will be at its lowest, you can really get to know what your infertile cervix feels like. And then in the next cycle you should check the cervix from day 6 onwards, or when your period finishes.

Unlike the cervical mucus method it is not necessary to check the cervix more than once a day. However, at the beginning, it can be instructive to check twice a day and you may be able to pick up changes in the course of the day. In fact there is a small *daily* variation in position of the cervix: it is very slightly lower towards the end of the day. For this reason it is important to check it at about the same time, preferably later in the day.

Softening. Around ovulation the cervix softens — with a texture

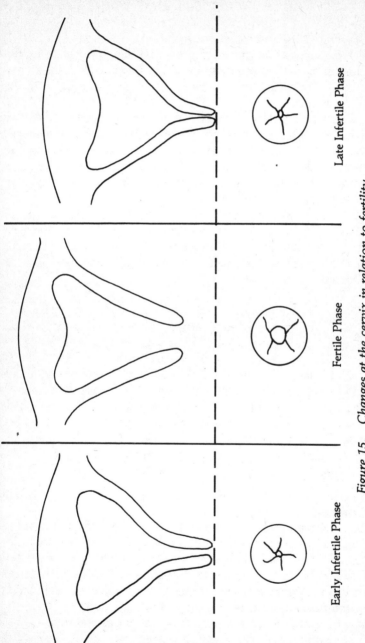

Early Infertile Phase   Fertile Phase   Late Infertile Phase

Figure 15.   Changes at the cervix in relation to fertility.

like your lower lip. At infertile times it is firmer, feeling like the tip of your nose.

Opening. The cervix is relatively closed off — sealed by a thick plug of mucus — the opening feeling like a dimple on infertile days. Close to ovulation, it opens, and at the height of fertility, it may admit the fingertip. If you have had children, the opening will be more slit-like.

You may find that this sign is the easiest to detect. The other changes are quite subtle differences from one day to the next requiring you to remember what the cervix was like on the previous day: your tactile memory tells that there has been a change, that the cervix is beginning to rise and soften, and therefore fertility is increasing.

Not all women appear to experience all these classic changes of the cervix. Indeed you may notice only one or two of these signs. And it may take three or more cycles to be confident about relying on these changes. Nonetheless, these cervical signs are well worth observing as a double-check.

Mucus. The value of detecting mucus directly at the cervix is that it can give you even earlier warning — sometimes a day or more — of impending ovulation. The spongy vaginal walls may slow down the descent of the early thicker, sticky mucus.

Note that vaginal walls are moist so that the examining fingers will be wet. At infertile times, the surface of the cervix will usually be slightly moist, but it can be dry and gritty. The more fertile mucus gives it a slippery wet feeling. In order to see this mucus, it can be helpful to 'milk' the cervix. Two fingers either side of the cervix are gently squeezed together and then withdrawn to the outside. Any mucus can then be stretched between the fingertips and observed.

Charting the cervix

The changes at the cervix can be represented on the chart as follows (see Figure 16). The infertile cervix is shown by a dot towards the lower end of the space to show that it is closed and low in position, and firmness by the abbreviation 'f'. As the fertile cervix rises and opens, it is represented by an enlarged circle higher in the space, and softening by s. Mucus can be marked in the same way as the quality of mucus that appears externally, but it is, of course, observed and noted separately in its own space on the chart.

Figure 16. Charting cervical changes.

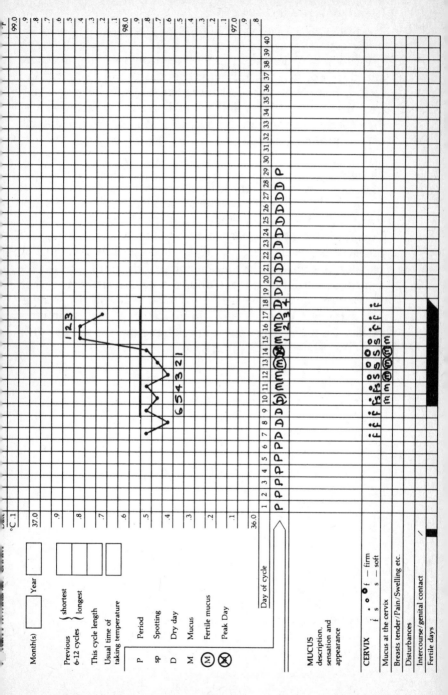

Conditions affecting the cervix

The principal ones are *cervical erosions* (see page 62) and *cancer of the cervix*.

Whilst cauterizing the cervix for an erosion is a minor procedure and does not permanently affect mucus production, cervical cancer has more serious consequences. The diagnosis and treatment is cone biopsy and, depending on how extensive it is, many of the mucus-producing 'glands' may be destroyed, making conception much less likely.

Summary

Many women find it very helpful to check the cervix. It is not an essential part of fertility awareness and it can take a little longer than the cervical mucus method to distinguish changes in fertility. You may find that one particular sign is more obvious than the others. Whichever change you first notice is the clue to your rising fertility, and this marks the beginning of the fertile phase. The return to infertility, once ovulation is over, is usually faster than the more gradual changes prior to ovulation. While temperature and external mucus are the main indicators of the late infertile phase, it is possible to double-check these signs with three days of a low, closed and firm cervix.

5.

The Art of Natural Birth Control

The key to successfully avoiding pregnancy by fertility awareness — as well as being clear about the techniques — is to know yourself! With artificial contraception, your participation is minimal. Nothing is required of you with the IUD, and with the Pill you just have to get into the habit of remembering to take it. Natural birth control, on the contrary, requires your full co-operation with what has been given — your fertility — and that you learn to read and respond to nature's signs. You are making the choice of controlling your own fertility, knowing that unprotected intercourse at fertile times may lead to pregnancy. This responsibility does not have to be a burden! While there are certain pitfalls to beware of, we shall also look at the benefits of natural birth control. *Art* implies putting everything in its right place. The art of natural birth control is to harmonize all aspects of fertility — spiritual, psychological and physical.

When you have observed one or two cycles, you may begin to notice how certain moods, feelings and changes in sensitivity correspond to your fertility cycle. *Some* women find that not only do they experience most sexual desire at the fertile time, but that it is quite indiscriminate! This can be an important observation to make, because you may find as a result that you get less tangled up in relationships you do not really want. Other women feel irritable and can hardly bear to be touched at this time. Surveys looking at the relationship of sexual desire to the female cycle show no constant pattern. Many women feel most interested in sex just before or just after the period. It is interesting to speculate why this lack of synchronization between biological fertility and desire should occur. It certainly implies there's more to sex than having babies — as if we hadn't suspected that. But there's also the factor that many of us neither expect or want to have child after child. Perhaps we intuitively know when we are fertile, much of the time? And so we condition ourselves to feel less sexual when we know pregnancy is likely?

Irrespective of the method of birth control you use, it has been shown that you are much more likely to make it work if you are certain you don't want a pregnancy, than if you envisage a child sometime in the near future. Your motivation is the overriding factor in natural birth control. Do you actually know what you want? Is your mind clear? If confusion or ambivalence reigns, sooner rather than later you will probably get pregnant. It is only too easy in this frame of mind — especially if you are not sure whether you are fertile or not — to assume that it is bound to be alright this month, after all last month you got away with it! Many women are very afraid of an unplanned pregnancy, and paradoxically it is this very fear which, unexamined, causes great confusion and leads to error.

Fertility awareness methods and the single woman

In this era of AIDS, if you are not in a long-term relationship, it makes sense to insist that your partner use a condom with care on every occasion of intercourse. The evidence is that this should substantially protect both of you, not only against HIV infection, but also against the other sexually-transmitted diseases which can have such a devastating effect on a woman's fertility.

There may well be a point when a relationship moves into a more committed phase. You might then consider — if you haven't done so already — the value of HIV antibody testing before allowing unprotected intercourse.

Sharing it with your partner

If you are in a long-term relationship, the decision to use natural birth control must be one made freely by both of you. It is not the method of choice for a couple who find it impossible to talk to each other! At the same time, using natural birth control can deepen your understanding of each other, and improve the quality of your relationship.

Since you are the one who has the fertility cycles, it may seem at first thought that there is little your partner can do to be involved in the process. However, at the very least he could, for example, read and shake down the thermometer and record your temperature on the chart. If he wants to understand more, and you have enough mucus, you could show him so that he sees the characteristic features of the mucus on which your combined fertility depends. Another thing he could do, especially if you find it difficult to reach your cervix, is check it for you.

An important aspect of a man's responsibility for natural birth control is to respect your fertility, and to develop a greater understanding of what it is to be affectionate and loving. There are, of course, three main options: to use a barrier method, practise coitus reservatus or to avoid intercourse at the fertile time. What you both decide to do, and how you cope with it, depends on a number of factors — personal, aesthetic and religious.

Avoiding intercourse

Some religions prohibit not only any intimate contact which does not lead to intercourse, but all forms of physical contact at certain times of the cycle. Such constraints do not have to block communication. You can still delight in each other's presence and express affection in ways other than sexual intercourse.

'Abstinence' is an unfortunate word. It conjures up such harsh denial in our minds. There seems to be nothing positive in it. In fact it often leads to a fundamental re-evaluation of experiences of sex and love. For example, it is sometimes the case that what we actually want is to be held, cuddled and loved, and not to have intercourse at all. On other occasions, sex becomes a way of relieving frustration and boredom, or of making up to each other after a row. And we often expect our partner to feel the same way about sex at the same time as us.

If you have decided not to have intercourse in the fertile phase, it can be a time to experiment with different ways of making love. It is a chance to be creative in love-making without the 'end-gaining' approach that habitual intercourse may bring! And when anything is possible again, there is often a feeling of freshness and renewal in making love once more.

Coitus reservatus

This book, when first printed, made the almost universal error of condemning and misrepresenting 'withdrawal'. The usual image of coitus interruptus is of the man belatedly pulling out and leaving his partner frustrated. What we are talking about, instead, is more properly and pompously called 'coitus reservatus'! This implies that the man allows his build-up of excitement to take place slowly. In doing so, he allows his partner to achieve her orgasm first. He must ensure he doesn't come anywhere near approaching orgasm whilst inside the vagina.

Now let us look at the evidence for the alleged shortcomings of 'withdrawal' (discussed in more detail in John Guillebaud's *Contraception*, and by Malcolm Potts, co-author with Peter Diggory, of *Textbook of Contraceptive Practice*). The few studies that have been carried out comparing the effectiveness of withdrawal with that of the diaphragm showed marginally better rates for withdrawal. The ~ssertion often made, that the pre-ejaculate contains sperm whic., would lead to pregnancy has not been proven either way.

If you *must avoid pregnancy at all costs* the advice is, whether you use coitus reservatus or barrier methods, to avoid intercourse on days of highly-fertile mucus — and for a couple of days after peak. Unprotected intercourse would then be restricted entirely to the post-ovulatory phase.

Using barrier methods

The use of barrier methods — in conjunction with fertility awareness methods — is generally disapproved of in natural family planning circles for moral reasons, often with claims about the impossibility of combining the two. Certainly it is true that spermicides used alone (not recommended), or with the diaphragm or cap, will obscure mucus *externally*. They will not, however, prevent you from obtaining and interpreting pristine mucus directly from the cervix. Even spermicidal-coated condoms should not interfere with external mucus observation.

Propositions about the 'un-naturalness' of barrier methods seem to us to founder on the fact of deliberate intent to avoid pregnancy, whatever the means employed.

Barrier methods can be used very successfully — and minimally — with the guidance of fertility awareness. They permit a flexibility of approach in the fertile phase of the cycle, sometimes the woman taking responsibility for contraception, sometimes the man. And in the early stages of using fertility awareness methods, until confidence is established in the pre-ovulatory phase, barrier methods can be a great asset.

It is a pity they have such a poor image. This is partly attributable to the circumstances in which they are first used: unsure of ourselves in our early sexual experiences; fumbling around in the dark for those condoms (where did I put them?) — rolling it on the wrong way while rapidly loosing an erection; the chilling trip to the bathroom for the diaphragm which has the unfortunate tendency to spring right out of your hand!

Why exclude barrier methods from your love-making? Eroticise them! — include them as part of your fore-play. If spermicides turn you off, consider that in Australia, family planning clinics are advising women not to bother using spermicides at all with the diaphragm. A trial is currently underway at the Margaret Pyke Centre in London to see whether the use of spermicides increases the effectiveness of the diaphragm. Can you believe it? — no-one has actually proved, in fifty years of their use — that it makes any difference! As far as condoms are concerned, if you object to the messiness of spermicidal-coated ones, non-spermicidal ones are, of course, available, as well as special allergy ones for those so afflicted. Condoms splitting in use (sharp fingernails excepted) are extremely rare, and the spermicidal veneer would only make a marginal difference in such an eventuality.

Now that we have discussed some of the human factors in natural birth control, we can consider how the various methods can be combined to avoid pregnancy.

6.

Natural Birth Control Guidelines

Starting out

If you have depended on artificial contraception in the past, it can seem a big step to trust your own body's fertility signs and your interpretation of them. If you have an IUD, you may prefer to continue with it in place until you are sure of understanding your fertility cycles. The only difficulties here are that, if you have prolonged bleeding, the beginning of the mucus build-up may be masked, and if you are having intercourse frequently, you will not be able to observe so clearly the changes in mucus from day to day. If you are on the Pill, the synthetic hormones block your fertility and its signs, so you will need, of course, to come off it (see page 61).

Your first aim in natural birth control should be to identify the beginning of the late infertile phase. If you start charting near the start of a cycle, and it is of average length, within two to three weeks you should be able to have unprotected intercourse following a clearly-defined temperature shift: that is, from the morning of the third consecutive higher temperature, all higher temperatures being above the level of the previous six; a rise of at least 0.2°C (0.4°F) between the last lower end and (one of) the three higher temperatures.

In the early part of the cycle, while you are learning the cervical mucus method, you will need to use condoms or abstain. Your second aim should be to identify peak day; and then the double-check guideline for the late infertile phase is as follows:

The late infertile phase begins once you have identified three higher temperatures after peak day.

Some authorities recommend going by whichever indicator comes *later*. This seems to us to ignore the contribution *each* indicator makes; and it may mean that you lose a day in the post-ovulatory phase which would be available for unprotected intercourse without any extra risk of pregnancy.

Let's now look at some examples of how this works in practice:

- temperature shift follows immediately after peak day: unprotected intercourse will be safe from the third *evening* after peak.

- temperature shift occurs before peak: still wait for three higher temperatures *after* peak (even if that means waiting for your fourth or fifth higher temperature after the shift.)

- temperature shift occurs as late as two days post-peak: you will be safe on the *morning* of the fourth day after peak.

Then the sky is the limit — you are free to have intercourse safely for the rest of the cycle!

You should find that, in most cycles, the temperature and mucus signs agree to within a couple of days of each other. Occasionally you may find that they are more than two days out of synchronization with each other. In trying to account for this discrepancy, when your cycle is complete, count back twelve to sixteen days from the first day of the following period. Then you can compare this calculated probable time of ovulation with your knowledge of the likely times of ovulation from the mucus and temperature records (see pages 24 and 34). If this is still a problem, it would be best to consult a teacher of NFP.

The true period rule

In the first cycle you chart, you will know when to expect your period — approximately ten days after the third higher temperature.

The first six days of the next cycle will be infertile in most circumstances. So the length of time for unrestricted intercourse can be extended from the late infertile phase of one cycle through the first six days of the next cycle. There are three conditions applying to this rule:

1. A temperature shift previously implies that any subsequent bleeding must be a true menstruation.
2. Cycles should not regularly tend to be very short in length (twenty-four days or less).
3. No signs of mucus.

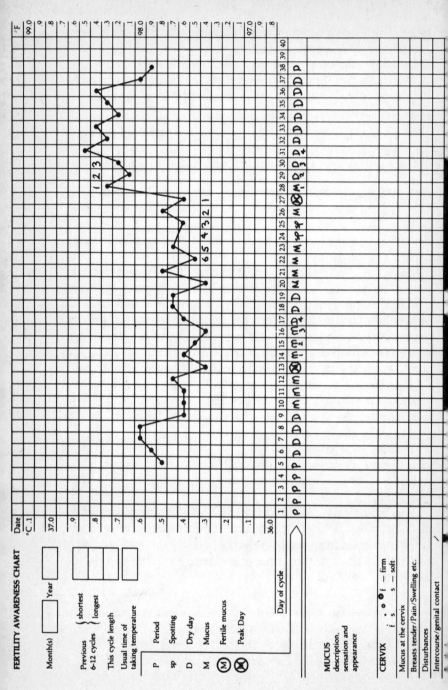

Figure 17. Ovulation bleeding is not menstruation.

You may have heard panic stories about women getting pregnant by having intercourse during their period! What is the explanation for this? One possibility is that ovulation bleeding may be mistaken for the onset of menstruation, especially in a longer-than-usual cycle (see Figure 17). The other explanation is that if a cycle is extremely short and menstruation prolonged, it is possible that early mucus may be masked by continued bleeding.

There is no evidence that pregnancy has ever resulted from intercourse prior to the fourth day of the cycle. Therefore, if your cycles are especially short, you can only assume that the first four days are infertile.

As soon as the period ends, you must be on the alert for the earliest signs of mucus. This may only be a change from a positive feeling of nothingness to one of being no longer dry, rather than actually being able to see mucus (or, with great care, the change from a continuous background mucus to fertile mucus). Until then, the early day rule applies, according to the Billings method.

Is the early day rule strictly necessary?

Intercourse is only advised on *alternate evenings* in the early infertile phase following the period, according to them. They further advise that intercourse should be restricted to the *evenings*, because only then will gravity have given any mucus produced an opportunity to appear externally. And it applies to alternate days because following intercourse, seminal fluid and vaginal secretions may mask any mucus that appears for a variable number of hours afterwards. It is often summarized by:

'Dry day, safe night, skip a day.'

Of course, once you are able to include checking the cervix, you are neither limited to alternate days, nor evenings.

The fertile phase begins with the earliest sign of mucus, double-checked by the cervix whichever comes FIRST. Most women find it takes two to six cycles before they are confident enough to go beyond day 6 of the cycle.

On page 17 we discussed some of the reasons for the failure of the rhythm method. It is with the greatest reluctance that we include any detail of calendar calculations. They are still taught in mainstream NFP as a double-check against mucus, especially if the cervix is not examined. We no longer believe in recommending any calendar calculations. They encourage women to 'think rhythm' and therefore discount their own observations; and the calculation usually prohibits any unprotected intercourse beyond day 6 of the cycle anyway. That being said, for your interest, the basis of the rhythm method in determining the beginning of the fertile phase (by knowing the shortest length of your previous six to twelve cycles) is as follows:

Shortest cycle minus 18 days = first day of fertile phase.

For example, if your shortest cycle in the previous 6 to 12 was 25 days, then day 7 is the first unsafe fertile day (that is, day 6 is the last day on which you would have intercourse). Even if you have only just started observing your fertility cycles, you may have kept a note of your periods, and so you will be able to calculate the shortest cycle.

The reason for the *minus 18 rule* is to allow for the earliest possible ovulation — 16 days before the next period — and three days' sperm survival. This double-check method maintains a possible effectiveness of about 97 per cent. If you are very anxious about the need to avoid pregnancy, you may push the method effectiveness close to 99 per cent by using a calculation of S (shortest cycle) minus 20: this allows for sperm survival extended to five days. (You may also come across a calculation S-21: this refers to the *last safe day*, and so comes to the same as the S-20 formula.) Some authorities suggest a compromise, following a S-19 rule.

There is also a calendar calculation based on the temperature method and the previous six to twelve cycles. This was used in the days before mucus was known about and gave a surprisingly high degree of method effectiveness (with twelve cycles), comparable to that of the compromise S-19 formula above. It is:

Day of first higher temperature of the shortest cycle minus six days = first fertile day.

For example, if day 14 was the earliest day of temperature rise, then from day 8 onwards it would be unsafe for intercourse.

If you are prepared to accept a method-effectiveness of 97%, then you can rely on mucus alone; if you add in checking the cervix, you should be able to achieve an even higher effectiveness. If the *highest* degree of safety is required, only rely on the post-ovulatory phase and the first four days of the next cycle (that is still about fourteen days available for unprotected intercourse).

Finding your way

You now have all the basic information needed to practice natural birth control successfully. When you have a little experience, you will know which method or combination of methods suits you best. And it won't be necessary to observe every day of your cycle, unless you prefer to stick to a routine.

Using the temperature method, you do not need to begin temperature recording until the mucus build-up starts — it usually takes six days or more. (However, if your cycles tend to be very short, you must start recording from day 5 onwards in order to take six lower temperatures.) Once you are in the late infertile phase, you can drop recording temperature and mucus altogether. The only time when you would need to resume temperature-taking again would be if your period did not come when expected. If your temperature was still up twenty days after the rise, you would most probably be pregnant.

7.

Changing Patterns

The rhythm method was hopeless in dealing with irregular or prolonged cycles, and with the changing patterns following the Pill, childbirth and approaching the menopause. In these circumstances, if you observe mucus which does not change in character or amount for two weeks, you have positively identified an infertile pattern of mucus. It is practically impossible to have fertile mucus for as long as two weeks. You then carefully watch for any departure from this basic infertile pattern which signifies rising fertility. In the meantime you must follow the early day rule unless you are checking the cervix as well. The last day of this changing, more fertile mucus is peak day. The late infertile phase begins, as usual, on the evening of the third higher temperature after peak — or on the fourth evening if you are going by mucus alone.

It is not so easy, however, when the underlying hormone pattern is unstable or in transition. As the body tries to ovulate, there may be recurrent patches of more fertile mucus. Just when you're clear of one patch, another one appears. This may seem confusing and frustrating, especially if NFP is new to you and you have not observed the changes in fertility in more regular circumstances. But your body's signs will clearly indicate what is happening. It will be a time when your priorities are questioned. If you are prepared to patiently make your observations from day to day, you will soon learn to recognize your state of fertility. You then have to decide whether or not you are going to use a barrier method at certain times, or for a longer period of time, or not at all.

It will be of great help to go by cervix and temperature as well as external mucus. The temperature shift will tell you which patch of fertile mucus corresponded with ovulation, and that you can therefore expect your period soon. The cervical signs will support your external mucus observations and give you added confidence.

We will now examine how to apply fertility awareness to these changing patterns.

The aftermath of the Pill
Unwanted effects of the Pill are not uncommon and range from the fairly trivial to the very serious and even death. There are other consequences, not well documented because they are not so *objective*, which are nonetheless vital to your well-being. The fact is that the Pill is a massive interference with the normal processes of the body, however much the dose of oestrogen is reduced or the mix of hormones tailored to the body's usual pattern.

How the Pill works
The combined and triphasic Pills — which contain synthetic oestrogen and progestogen — work by blocking ovulation, making the cervical mucus hostile to sperm and impairing the lining of the womb. This happens by the suppression of the centres which naturally regulate oestrogen and progesterone produced in the ovaries.

The 'Mini-Pill' contains progestogen only. It affects the mucus and the womb, but it does not always inhibit ovulation, in which case it may interfere with the implantation of an already fertilized egg.

With this intimate disturbance of functioning, it is not surprising that some women coming off the Pill realize that once more they *feel themselves*. The body may tolerate interference for years yet if the Pill is re-started, a severe reaction against it can take place.

Fertility awareness post-Pill
While you are on the Pill you cannot — of course — observe the physical changes accompanying your own hormonal cycle which are suppressed by the synthetic hormones. You should wait until you have finished taking the Pill for that 'cycle'. There will be a withdrawal bleed — not a true period — a few days later. You can date the beginning of your first cycle after the Pill from the first day of bleeding.

How soon your cycles return to normal varies. There may be no apparent consequences of being on the Pill. Alternatively, you may notice you have one or two anovulatory cycles; or ovulation may be delayed, usually for no more than two months. In the meantime you may experience a continuous discharge of fertile-like mucus. This is thought to be caused by the release of synthetic oestrogen stored in fatty tissue in the body.

Another reason for an abnormal amount of mucus is the presence of a *cervical erosion* (which is also common after pregnancy). This is a condition where the lining of the cervical canal grows out over the opening of the cervix, and it has a red raw appearance. The area affected can be cauterized if the discharge is a nuisance, although most erosions will resolve spontaneously if left alone. You can expect an abnormally thin discharge for approximately two weeks afterwards. If a larger area has to be treated the quantity of mucus may be affected, but its quality and timing will not be.

The other post-Pill effect to be aware of is a shortening of the post-ovulatory phase in the first two or three cycles.

Ideally you should wait for a couple of months before trying for a baby. This gives your body time to revert to its natural hormone balance and for you to practice good pre-pregnancy care. Should you become pregnant during this time there is no harm to the baby. Especially if this is your first experience of fertility awareness, it is preferable not to resume unprotected intercourse until you are definitely in the late infertile phase of the cycle. Wait until the morning of the fourth higher temperature — or the evening of the third higher temperature, if you have identified peak day. If it looks as though ovulation will be significantly delayed, you may prefer to use a barried method in this period.

The only other likely problem is a yeast infection ('thrush'), which needs to be taken care of (see page 41). Within a short time, you should be experiencing normal cycles and easily identifying your fertility patterns.

Following childbirth

Many women and their partners review their choice of contraceptive method at this time. Unfortunately, especially if there has been no previous experience of charting, it is probably the hardest time to learn fertility awareness methods, and most couples would be better served by barrier methods. For those who are highly motivated to make it work, or for those who wish to monitor their returning fertility, there follows a basic account of what to expect.

Immediately after your baby is born there is no need to do anything about birth control, and it is the last thing you want to think about at such a special time! If you can breastfeed, preferably for at least some months, you will give your baby a wonderful start in life; physically and emotionally you both benefit. La Leche League offers experienced help if you have any questions or difficulty breastfeeding, and they also have a wide range of literature on this and related subjects (see Useful Addresses).

The earliest that ovulation can return is 43 days after the birth when you are totally and solely breastfeeding: that is, 'demand feeding', with the breast as the pacifier; the baby has no solids and breastfeeds during the night as well. In this way, there are less than a few hours between feeds. Repeated suckling at the breast stimulates the release of the hormone *prolactin* from the pituitary gland, producing milk, and inhibiting oestrogen. Therefore the characteristic mucus build-up and ovulation is suppressed for some time, often a year or more.

On the other hand, 'partial' breastfeeding, with longer intervals between feeds (for example, the baby sleeps all the way through the night), may not delay ovulation any longer than bottlefeeding. It can occur as early as *four weeks* after birth. (In the world as a whole, breastfeeding — and malnutrition — are the main regulators of birth, more important than artificial contraception, and so the policy of certain multi-national companies in promoting substitute milks in the underdeveloped world is deplorable.)

The other important point about returning fertility after childbirth is that you cannot rely on the return of periods to give you sufficient warning of your first ovulation. In a substantial minority of women, ovulation takes place before the first period.

The basic infertile pattern
After the lochia (the blood-stained discharge following childbirth) clears up, you may have days or weeks of dryness and no mucus at all. The early day rule applies unless you are double-checking with the cervix.

If you are bottlefeeding, or only partially breastfeeding, you must start charting three weeks after birth. Otherwise you need not begin until you first notice mucus, or after nine weeks. You should not assume that this mucus is infertile until you have observed its unchanging pattern for two weeks. It may be thick and sticky, or flaky and crumbly, or thin and wet or milky. This may seem a bit strange if you have observed mucus before, where the interpretations 'fertile' and 'less fertile' were quite clearly applied to a specific kind of mucus: now we are emphasizing the *unchanging* pattern of the mucus.

As soon as there is any sign of change in amount, or to a stretchy mucus with some 'body', or there is a lubricative wet sensation, you must assume that you are fertile. The last day of altered mucus is designated 'peak', and it will be safe to resume intercourse on the fourth evening afterwards.

Daily checking of the cervix for signs of ripening or the early appearance of mucus will give you added confidence in trusting your basic infertile pattern, especially if you have never observed the normal changes in mucus before. It is not necessary to chart temperature at this stage. You may be in for many months of infertility and disturbed nights' sleep.

Prolonged breastfeeding and continually low oestrogen levels may occasionally cause the vagina to dry out and produce a discharge which is thin, grey and watery but is not lubricative or stretchy.

The transition phase
It is fairly straight-forward to use natural birth control while you are in a stable infertile state. Shortly before your cycles return, 'attempts' are made to ovulate. Patches of fertile mucus begin to appear — more and more frequently — without ovulation actually occurring.

You should begin temperature-taking, then, as soon as you begin to notice fertile mucus, or your baby starts to sleep through the night, take solids or breastfeed less. If you are having very disturbed nights — perhaps with other young children as well — and your temperature record is all over the place, it is worth trying to take your temperature at a regular time just before you go to bed — say 10 p.m. This will sometimes produce a more settled chart, which should follow fairly closely the pattern of basal body temperature recording.

The temperature record will tell you which episode of fertile mucus is linked with ovulation. Any spotting of blood or actual bleeding should not be assumed as menstruation unless preceded by a clear temperature rise. If you look carefully, you may notice that such ovulatory bleeding is accompanied by fertile mucus.

The effect of stress during breastfeeding — unlike normal circumstances — is to allow ovulation to occur *earlier* than it might otherwise. Prolactin is inhibited, oestrogen levels creep up, and fertile cycles return much sooner. It is important to rest as much as possible and to eat nourishing food; breastfeeding is more demanding of nutrients than pregnancy itself.

This change-over from infertility to fertility is perhaps the most difficult time to learn and apply fertility awareness. It is particularly helpful to ask for the guidance of a teacher or a woman who has used natural birth control at this time herself. Depending on how long weaning takes, you may want to use a barrier method of birth control until your periods return.

The first few cycles
When your periods return, you will probably find that it takes a few months for your cycles to settle down again. These early cycles are likely to be less fertile and of variable length. If ovulation occurs, it may be followed by menstruation after a shorter interval than will be usual.

Your fertile mucus now may not be so very different from the 'infertile' mucus you experienced while breastfeeding. This is because, while breastfeeding, the character of the mucus depends on the balance between prolactin and the ovarian hormones while, in normal circumstances, the balance is between the ovarian hormones oestrogen and progesterone. If you want to use an accurate calendar calculation as a double-check for the beginning of the fertile phase, you must start counting six to twelve cycles again.

Approaching the menopause
The 'change of life' is the winding down of fertility and its accompanying psychological and hormonal readjustments. Sometimes periods just stop. Usually, however, there is a gradual decline in fertility. The ovarian hormones oestrogen and progesterone are secreted less frequently and in smaller amounts. It takes about two to three years for the adrenal glands to take over producing a baseline level of oestrogen. In the meantime the action of the male hormone testosterone, of which small amounts are present, is unopposed by oestrogen, and may contribute to feelings of irritability and aggression. Eventually no more progesterone is produced at all.

It is also the time of many changes psychologically. Children grow up and leave home. Your own parents are growing old or have died. Perhaps you start to look back over your life and wonder again about its purpose. There may be the fear of a late

pregnancy and its consequences — including the increased risk
of a child born with Down's syndrome (Mongolism).

In fact the risk of pregnancy over the age of 45 is extremely
low *without* birth control measures. Over 50 there is an
infinitesimally small risk. Moreover, by understanding fertility
awareness you will be able to identify any days of possible fertility.

Cycle changes

Cycles that were formerly regular become variable in length. If
you were used to using rhythm calculations you may find they
are now of no use at all. Some cycles can be very short. It is
advisable not to *assume* infertility beyond day 4 of the cycle
(compared with day 6 in normal circumstances) — preceded of
course by a temperature shift. In the course of the longer ones
it is important not to lose patience with daily observation and
charting. Otherwise you may have intercourse during an
unexpectedly late fertile phase.

Vaginal bleeding

You may notice more bleeding in the course of the cycle. When
this happens just before, and merging into, the menstrual flow,
it is caused by progesterone levels being too low to maintain the
lining of the uterus. It is sometimes difficult to decide exactly when
the next cycle begins. In these circumstances, as a rough guide,
you can date the first day of the new cycle from when the
temperature drops.

Spotting, or several days of bleeding, occurring earlier in the
cycle may be ovulation bleeding and you must assume this. You
then wait until three higher temperatures past the last day of this
bleeding, or the fourth evening if you notice mucus unmasked
by the bleeding.

Mucus patterns

Mucus appearing at this time of life is typically scanty, and may
be thick and sticky or crumbly and flaky. If it is unchanging —
and this fact will be established over a couple of weeks'
observation — then it constitutes the basic infertile pattern.
Sometimes there may only be a day or so of fertile mucus
appearing at the outside: the cervix can be a useful double-check.

In some cycles there may be a temperature rise, and yet no
fertile mucus is produced. These will be infertile, although

ovulation occurs, because of the absence of the mucus necessary to sustain and transport the sperm.

As oestrogen levels fall, there may be a number of disturbing effects, including episodes of hot flushes and breast soreness. The lining of the vagina may become dry and intercourse painful: this can be alleviated by KY jelly or by local hormone creams.

The number of cycles in which ovulation occurs, decrease. Eventually menstruation ceases. When more than a year has elapsed since your last period you are said to have reached the menopause, but it may be worthwhile to continue charting for a further six months to be absolutely sure.

Hormone replacement therapy (HRT)
It seems the obvious thing to replace the hormones that are low and apparently causing problems. However, there are at least two good arguments against this. The action of synthetic hormones may delay the natural process of the change of life, so that you have to go through it when you stop taking the tablets. Secondly, there are serious hazards associated with HRT, including an increased incidence of cancer of the uterus and breast. So you should consider carefully whether possible temporary relief of symptoms (and it is thought the placebo effect may be large part of it) is worth the considerable dangers of long-term use. Is the change of life an illness requiring treatment? Or is it an opportunity to learn about loss and change and renewal?

8.

Preparing for Pregnancy

Having a baby should bring great joy, but it can be a mixed blessing. Being aware of your state of fertility from day to day, and knowing that intercourse at the fruitful time of the cycle is likely to lead to pregnancy, brings you face to face with the possible consequences to you and your unborn child if pregnancy is unwanted.

It is not something to be afraid of — the only 100 per cent method of birth control is total abstinence! So, living close to the edge demands that you know what you want. If you want a child, what are your reasons? What do you hope it might bring to your relationship? Are you going to have a child because you think you should — for example, to please your partner? If you are single, how do you see rearing a child on your own? What is the kind of security a child needs to happily grow and fulfill its potential as a human being? These are surely questions to which only you can find the answers.

To bring a new life into this world, and all it implies, is not a casual thing. Does it make having a baby sound rather worked out and not the spontaneous act some people think it 'ought' to be? On the contrary, if you are clear in your mind as to what you must do, making love at the fertile time does not mean you have to become self-conscious about it.

Before that time, though, you and your partner have a responsibility to be as healthy as possible. Pregnancy, childbirth and your child will place great demands on both of you which will have to be met.

Nutrition is an important factor. A varied wholefood diet, low in processed and animal foods, should supply the nourishment needed without overloading the body. And it is worth learning the art of cooking: 'healthy' meals can be very tasty.

Both of you should have health screening. Has there been any recent exposure to drugs, medicines or chemicals? It is important for the woman to check her rubella (German measles) status: infection early in pregnancy can have disastrous consequences for the proper development of the baby.

If you have just had a coil taken out, it is probably worth waiting until your periods return to normal. That should give a good indication that the lining of the womb has healed. As mentioned before, ideally you should wait for a couple of months after coming off the Pill before trying for a baby. As well as needing the time to recover from the derangement of your normal hormone balance, you probably will have very little idea of when you conceived unless you practise fertility awareness.

Some women just *know* when they conceive. This is often dismissed by doctors on the grounds of being too subjective! When you have had higher temperatures for twenty days, then you can show objective evidence that you are pregnant. If you have been observing mucus as well, and you can remember when you made love, it is possible to conclude to within a day or so either side your probable date of conception.

Estimating the date of birth

There is an average time from conception to birth of 266 days (38 weeks): the range is ± 2 weeks in 90 per cent of women. By the traditional method of counting from the first day of the last period, the duration of pregnancy is reckoned to be 280 days (40 weeks). The simple calculation your doctor uses holds well in average-length cycles. The time of birth is:

First day of last period plus 7 days plus 9 calendar months.

For example, if your last period began on 6 January, your baby would be born about 13 October.

This calculation falls down when the cycle in which conception occurred is a long one. The formula can then be modified as follows:

Day of peak or temperature rise minus 7 days plus 9 calendar months.

Had the temperature risen on 3 February in the previous example, the baby would be expected around 27 October — two weeks later than the traditional formula would give. Of course an ultrasound scan would also give information about the maturity of

The baby, but, again, only from an average point of view. So your baby is potentially in more danger of being induced unnecessarily unless you know yourself when you conceived. That way there is more chance that your baby will be allowed to come into the world when he is ready.

Choosing the sex of your baby?
There is a theory that the 'male' sperm (carrying Y chromosomes) swim faster and die quicker than the larger X-bearing 'female' sperm. Hence, if you want a girl, make love at the beginning of the fertile time, and if it's a boy you're after, try close to peak.

This theory is a very attractive one, but there is no good evidence testifying to its effectiveness. You have nothing to lose by trying it, but don't be disappointed if it doesn't work.

9.

Difficulty in Conceiving

Most couples who know about fertility awareness will achieve pregnancy in the first two or three cycles. If you haven't got pregnant after a year of trying, there may be a problem with you, your partner's, or your combined fertility: about fifteen per cent of couples have trouble conceiving. It is often a very complex situation, far beyond the scope of this book, but there are a number of excellent books on the subject if you want further information (see Further Reading, page 91).

The value of fertility awareness is that it enables you to do a great deal before you and your partner need undergo medical investigation. Available from chemists now are various home-testing kits which predict ovulation. You should consider their expense and the fact that they do not tell you anything more than your own observations.

Temperature recording
By keeping temperature charts, you can find out whether you are ovulating regularly. You can also see if the last part of the cycle is long enough for pregnancy to be established.

It takes at least six days for the egg, fertilized in the outer part of the fallopian tube, to travel down and implant in the lining of the womb (see Figure 10, page 33). After ovulation, a *corpus luteum* (which means 'yellow body' from its microscopic appearance) is formed on the surface of the ovary from where the egg has burst out. It produces progesterone which prepares the womb for the fertilized egg. The cervix closes and the mucus thickens so that the womb is sealed off from the outside world. The lining softens in order that the fertilized egg can embed in it. Body temperature rises and may have an incubating effect on the growth of the developing embryo.

If, however, the corpus luteum is not sustained, the *luteal phase* will be too short. The period will come within nine days of the temperature rise, implantation will be disturbed and such a cycle will be infertile.

Many doctors still recommend you *only* to take your temperature. From this you are expected to predict the most fertile time. As you know by now, the temperature shift cannot be as efficient as mucus and the cervix at indicating *at the time* your maximum fertility.

Timing intercourse

To summarize: the time to have intercourse is when you have fertile mucus, and as close to peak as possible; or, when the cervix is high, open and soft. The least efficient method is to time intercourse two to three days before and up to the expected temperature shift.

If you rarely ovulate and have long cycles and only a day or so (or a few hours) of fertile mucus, it can be easy to miss the fertile times altogether. And if there is very little mucus, you must be on the alert for a transient sensation of wetness.

It used to be advised that, if there was problem with the man's sperm-count, you should avoid intercourse for a few days to allow their numbers to build up. It now appears that this just allows an increase in the amount of geriatric and otherwise unfit sperm — not in the numbers of sperm in prime condition! It also tended to make intercourse seem very premeditated and fraught if there was a lot of anxiety about getting pregnant. In this situation it is better to forget about charting for a while.

The next step

By this time, if you still have not got pregnant, both of you should go to see what medical investigation may be needed. Don't forget to take your charts along!

One of the earliest investigations will be a *post-coital test*. This involves having a sample of mucus taken from your cervix after intercourse. The sample is examined under the microscope to see how your partner's sperm fare in your mucus. Antibodies are sometimes produced to the sperm, which are therefore destroyed.

Even when full investigations have been carried out, there may be no obvious reason why you cannot get pregnant. You may give up all hope of having a child, adopt one and then, very occasionally, it happens that pregnancy occurs! Acupuncture or

homoeopathy sometimes appears to make all the difference too.
Life works in mysterious ways!

10.

The Development of NFP

The story of NFP takes us on a fascinating journey through changing religious beliefs and secular attitudes towards sexuality and birth control, as well as through the development in scientific understanding of human fertility and its control. Here we trace a few of the main themes in recorded history, and then look to the future of NFP.

In many traditional cultures it was forbidden to have intercourse with a menstruating woman; abstinence was practised because of ancient taboos, for religious reasons and in attempts to regulate the birth-rate.

In the Bible, it is stated that 'when a woman has her menstrual flow, she shall be in a state of impurity for seven days' (Leviticus 15:19). And so, according to orthodox Judaism, a woman is 'unclean' for the whole of this time, at the end of which she must take a ritual purification bath in order that she can be touched once more by her husband. The injunction (Genesis 1:28) '. . . God said unto them, Be fruitful and multiply . . .' was expected to be fulfilled in Jewish Law, and shows a remarkable understanding of fertility awareness.

In Judaism, marriage is seen not as a matter of personal choice, but of religious duty: intercourse is the husband's responsibility and the wife's conjugal right. The use of contraception is sanctioned only for health reasons and must not interfere with the man's sperm. Procreation within marriage is even more important than the marriage itself. The sin of Onan was probably not masturbation (also strongly condemned), but coitus interruptus ('withdrawal') — when he spilt his seed on the ground in order to avoid impregnating the wife of his dead brother.

While Judaism recognizes the legitimacy of sexual pleasure in the aim of procreation, *early* Christianity sought to deny pleasure of all kind and to make chastity the supreme virtue. Confronted with the practical impossibility of trying to control all desire, the Church, while maintaining that sex outside of marriage was a mortal sin, conceded that between man and wife it could always be forgiven. (The best marriage, though, was metaphorically to Jesus and later the Church.)

The next step was to acknowledge the reality of procreation and so to approve of sexual intercourse within marriage, although the pleasure aspect was still suspect. Nevertheless, in the nineteenth century the Vatican gave Catholics permission to use periodic abstinence as a means of birth control. What was actually recommended was based on the theory of a French scientist that woman was fertile at the time of menstruation (equivalent to being 'on heat' in animals) and infertile the rest of the time. This method of natural birth control, called 'paternal prudence', must soon have given way to maternal mistrust!

Until recent times, disease, malnutrition and war limited the growth of the world's population and there was little political impetus for developing methods of birth control. In Victorian England, increasing numbers of women went out to work and the natural child-spacing effect of prolonged breastfeeding was lost. In addition, progress in public health meant that more babies survived infancy and into childhood.

Birth control was an idea whose time was coming. Introduction of early forms of the diaphragm and cap in the 1880s contributed to the emancipation of some women by giving them reliable control of their own fertility for the first time. The only method generally available was withdrawal, which, like barrier methods, was not permitted by the Church.

The availability for all of reliable birth control (in the developed world) is now taken for granted. It is salutary to understand something of the struggle which took place for the provision of family planning services in Britain.

At the turn of this century, public discussion of birth control took place in intellectual circles philosophizing about the need to balance food supply and population, and hardly at all about any benefit it might bring to the lives of ordinary men and women. In 1926, when the topic was mentioned in passing in a BBC discussion programme, an apology was broadcast because it had not been authorized. This was seven years after Marie Stopes' book *Married Love* had begun to stimulate public discussion on birth control. By 1921, she had set up two clinics in London, but, owing to strong disapproval, their function had to be concealed (one of them was called the 'Centre for Pre-Maternity and Child Welfare').

The 1930s saw the creation of a 'National Birth Control Council' (later to become the Family Planning Association) whose aim was to promote the setting up of clinics for *married women on health grounds*. Church doctrine on birth control divided: Protestants, with some reluctance, concluded it to be a matter of individual conscience and choice; Catholics adhered to the view that contraception is immoral and that the primary purpose of sex is procreation, but by the 1960s (and in more recent papal documents) sex had come to be seen in itself as a 'unifying and enriching factor' in marriage.

In 1967, twenty years after the National Health Service was set up, an Act was passed extending birth control facilities to the unmarried as well, and in 1974 the service was made completely free.

In the fourth century St Augustine (in his *Confessions*) had said: 'I was bound down by the disease of the flesh that only you [God] can cure'. Now, in our age of 'scientific enlightenment', we have moved from St Augustine's view of desire as disease to the assertion by a professor of psychiatry and sexologist that: 'inadequate sexual desire [is] probably the most pervasive of the sexual dysfunctions' (Helen Singer Kaplan, 1977).

The domination of the theologians has been taken over by the so-called experts in matters sexual — the sexologists. From the eighteenth century until well into this century, the idea of 'masturbatory insanity' held sway. This of course was fuelled by religious doctrine, but it had a powerful effect on popular beliefs. Masturbation came to be regarded both as a disease in itself, and a cause of diseases. Now the opposite view is held. Not to masturbate is a disease, and masturbation is recommended as treatment for the inability of a woman to have orgasmic intercourse. In the midst of such confusion, it is hardly surprising that there should still be considerable controversy over what should be taught in schools under the name of sex education. And so elementary facts of human biology — the signs of fertility — get lost in the ideological sex battle. Since fertility awareness is not taught in schools, who does teach it?

According to British government figures, it appears that in 1980 only 200 women were taught natural birth control methods on their first visit to a family planning clinic (compared with over

750,000 who went on the Pill). Yet from surveys of the British population, about 200,000 actually use natural birth control (and over 3 million the Pill). Even allowing for the fact that there are two main organizations that teach NFP and train teachers (Birmingham NFP Centre and the NFP Service of the Catholic Marriage Advisory Council), many women must have taught themselves or been taught by friends. While this is a very healthy sign, it does raise a question about the general quality of instruction — fertility awareness must be properly learnt. One does hear horror stories about pregnancies with NFP — as if the methods are only to blame: when an 'unwanted' pregnancy occurs, it is nearly always a problem of motivation or inadequate knowledge or understanding.

Were it not for the effects of, in the main, Catholic doctors and researchers to find acceptable methods of birth control for the faithful, it is probably the case that many of us would not now be able to avail ourselves of this knowledge for health or other reasons.

Many doctors and family planning staff actively discourage women from using NFP. Reasons for this are probably ignorance, pressure of time and the belief that women are not intelligent enough to take responsibility for themselves. A woman we taught had previously been to a well-known family planning clinic because she mistakenly thought that she would receive advice on getting pregnant — she was sent away in tears clutching a diaphragm.

Why has the women's movement, especially in Britain, not given more support to the growth of fertility awareness? One possibility is that they, as much as everyone else, still believe it is to do with the unacceptability of the rhythm method. Another factor is women's new sense of autonomy. The Pill and the IUD came to be seen as conveniences by which women could take control of their sexuality. The attempt to usurp the function of (male) doctors led to an obsession with the speculum and self-examination which alienated the majority of women who might otherwise have felt more inclined to participate in the relatively simple methods of fertility awareness.

Who should teach fertility awareness?
We believe it should be taught by people using NFP themselves. This is because its successful application depends on people who *know* and *trust* the methods they use. We were contacted by a

doctor who wanted further information so that she could teach NFP at one of her clinic sessions. It came up in the conversation that her method of birth control was the IUD. When we asked her why she did not use natural methods herself, she replied that she had three children and did not want another one!

If the teachers use NFP themselves, it is likely that there will be a strong grass-roots movement in NFP. The main hope for NFP lies in women helping each other cultivate their awareness *and* staying in touch with current scientific knowledge of NFP. If it only stays on an informal and casual level — and the situation now is that most teachers are volunteers, paid a token amount — then the general standard of instruction will suffer.

Teaching NFP

Curricula have been developed to standardize teaching. This is a step in the right direction but it can become too rigid. What is important in the end is not a slight difference in methods but a thorough understanding of the reasons for them, so that teaching can be adapted to suit specific situations.

As well as teaching individuals and couples, we also teach small group classes. This has the advantages for the client in providing a broader and often deeper experience learning how others see NFP and the sense that she is not entirely an odd-ball! For the teacher, there is an economizing of time and the effort in repeating the factual aspects of NFP: it is also a good deal of fun and very stimulating.

The future of NFP

The application of new technology to the problem of monitoring the fertility cycle has lead so far to the development of RITE TIME. This is an electronic fertility thermometer with a microprocessor which stores and computes the basal body temperature shift, thus avoiding the need for charting.

Because the *total* pregnancy rates for natural methods are higher than the Pill or IUD, the World Health Organization (1980) recommend that the main focus of research should be on developing new methods for identifying the fertile period. The hope is that this might lead to a reduction in the length of the abstinence required and therefore make it easier to follow the guidelines.

The most promising research being undertaken is the *Boots-Celltech project* to develop a simple urine dip-stick home-testing kit. It is designed to be sensitive to changes in the oestrogen/progesterone ratio and to change colour appropriately in the fertile phase of the cycle.

So, for the foreseeable future, we are likely to remain with that subjective assessment — *your own experience!* In fact you can judge your fertility nearly as well as the most sophisticated and expensive hormone tests currently used.

We hope this book makes a contribution to the spread of NFP. Real growth will occur as more and more of us using NFP share this knowledge with others.

Appendix A
Effectiveness

There is much confusion about the effectiveness of natural birth control when compared with other methods. Here we summarize the main evidence. Our conclusion is that the methods themselves are as reliable as other forms of birth control. The scientific trials show that they are applied with varying degrees of success, depending on motivation.

First, let us look at the theoretical effectiveness of methods of birth control. This measure is sometimes called *ideal, biological* or *method* effectiveness. It describes what would happen, were the methods to be used properly. Tietze (1970) grouped all widely used contraceptive methods — drawing on data from a number of studies — according to their theoretical effectiveness. We have summarized and brought up-to-date his findings as follows:

Theoretical Effectiveness %	Method
>99	sterilisation/vasectomy, combined Pill, temperature
>97	IUD, Mini-Pill, cap/diaphragm, condom, cervical mucus, combined methods of NFP
90	spermicides, rhythm

A theoretical effectiveness of 99 per cent implies that, of 100 women using the method properly for a year, only one would get pregnant. The temperature method is ranked alongside the most effective of methods; cervical mucus and combined methods of NFP with highly effective methods of contraception, and rhythm with less effective methods.

The classical way of representing the effectiveness of methods of birth control is to differentiate between *method-* and *use-* effectiveness: that is, what actually happens in practice. The following table shows the *average* range of effectiveness of the different methods in actual use:

Number of women out of 100 who are likely to become pregnant in one year	Method
1 - 3	Pills
2 - 7	IUD
7 - 12	condom
11 - 17	cap/diaphragm
5 - 15	NFP

Note: Table modified from *Population Reports*, 1981.

This range of effectiveness reflects the prime importance of the *intentions* of the couple. Those who definitely do not want a pregnancy in the foreseeable future ('limiters') have the lower pregnancy rates, whereas those who intend to have a baby in a short while — but not just yet — ('spacers') fare with much higher pregnancy rates. It is noteworthy that critics of NFP invariably compare the worst use-effectiveness rates for NFP with the best ones for other forms of contraception!

Other factors include degree of satisfaction and experience. If you have not found the method that best suits you, there is less inclination to use it properly or to continue to use it. Many pregnancies occur when a method has been dropped and no decision reached about an alternative. Younger users do less well, and the length of time a method is used is also a factor (the best trials now measure *extended* use-effective compared with the older Pearl Index).

Pregnancies which are not due to the imperfections of the method have been labelled 'user failures'. This does not make it clear what has actually happened, and there has been the suggestion that in future they should be divided as far as possible into these categories: *teaching-related* (a failure at some stage in the learning process); *informed-choice* (the couple knew there was the risk of pregnancy, although their stated intention was to avoid it), and *unresolved*.

When methods of NFP are compared, in particular a single method — cervical mucus — versus a combination of methods, the total pregnancy rate is approximately double (10-20 per cent against 5-10 per cent, respectively). Why there should be such a difference in practice, when the method effectiveness is comparable, is not known. It may reflect the fact that you are more likely to believe two warnings, rather than one, about the risk of pregnancy.

So, in general, we believe that modern methods of NFP are equivalent in actual effectiveness to the barrier methods. If you are really prepared to make the methods work for you, you can achieve as high an effectiveness as with any other method of contraception (except the combined Pill).

Appendix B.
The Scientific Basis of NFP

The real beginning of NFP was around 1930 when two researchers (Ogino and Knaus) independently showed that ovulation occurs approximately two weeks before the following period. This made it possible to calculate the probable fertile time, and this became the calendar or rhythm method.

Temperature

The next major advance was when Ferin (1947) showed, in a series of forty-two couples, that a rise in temperature could be used to avoid conception. Changes in body temperature in the course of the cycle had been reported in the nineteenth century, but it was not until 1928 that Van de Welde associated the temperature rise with the activity of the corpus luteum and thus ovulation. Apparently a little-known Catholic priest called Hillebrand had devised a combined method of NFP, using Knaus calculations and the changes in body temperature outlined in Van de Welde's work, in 1935.

Vollman (1940) correlated the temperature shift with mid-cycle pain. He also suggested averaging all the daily readings in one cycle to establish a baseline above which the higher temperatures could be determined in the next cycle.

Barton and Wiesner (1945) carried out research on waking temperatures in relation to fertility, and observed, in a small series of women, that pregnancy did not result from insemination more than three days before or after the temperature rise. Holt (1960) and Marshall (1963) and others worked out reliable guidelines for defining the temperature shift.

Hilgers and Bailey (1980) concluded that the temperature shift in 95 per cent of sixty-six cycles they monitored occurred over a seven-day range — three days either side of the day of ovulation.

In the other 5 per cent, the range was over ten days.

Vollman (1977) reported on cycles in which only one act of intercourse had taken place. His findings were that in forty-three cycles in which conception took place, the earliest pregnancy resulted from intercourse nine days before the shift, thirty-eight conceptions took place between the sixth day prior to the shift to one day after, and the last four conceptions occurred on the day of the second highest temperature.

Cervical mucus

In the mid-nineteenth century, some changes in cervical mucus were described, including how its condition affected sperm transport. No further work was done until 1933, when Seguy and Simonet linked the rise in urinary oestrogen before ovulation to changes in cervical mucus. In the 1940s Viergiver and Pommerenke associated the quantity and viscosity of mucus with sperm penetrability and body temperature.

In 1964, Billings formulated the rules of what he called the Ovulation Method. This gives the impression that the main value of observing mucus is to detect ovulation, but from a practical point of view it is to define the limits of fertility — hence 'cervical mucus method'.

The hormonal basis of the cervical mucus method was demonstrated by Billings, Brown and Burger (1972) and confirmed by Flynn and Lynch (1976). Hilgers and others (1977) recommended that, with the cervical mucus method alone, infertility should not be assumed until the evening of the fourth day past peak (the original rule was from the morning of that day). In 1978, he showed that ovulation takes place on peak day plus or minus two days.

Cervix

In 1932, Latz and Reiner suggested touching the cervix to feel for mucus as an indication of fertility. Apparently it was not followed up until 1962 when Keefe described the changes that can be felt at the cervix. No data has yet been gathered on the reliability or ease of observation of the cervical changes, although it has been the experience of many teachers and users that it is very useful as a double-check of the external mucus sign.

Combined methods

Doering (1967) reported on a large series of patients who used temperature and a calendar calculation (day of temperature rise of shortest cycle minus six days). Cervical mucus was not used, yet the method effectiveness was 98.5 per cent.

Roetzer (1965 and later work) made two major contributions: firstly that the first six days of the cycle carry an exceedingly low risk of pregnancy; secondly that he defines the late infertile phase as beginning on the evening of the third higher temperature after peak day. Beyond the first six days, he advises the observation of mucus and a calendar calculation of S-20 (which gives the last infertile day).

The Kippleys have written the most comprehensive guide to NFP to date from a Catholic viewpoint (*The Art of Natural Family Planning*, 1979). We are indebted to Thyma for his concept of the 'double-check'.

Appendix C
The Hormone Cycle

The hormonal system is a wonderfully balanced interplay of chemical responses and nerve impulses influencing and being affected by emotional states. We shall now try to summarize how it all fits together.

The main reproductive hormones oestrogen and progesterone are linked by a feed-back process with hormones from the anterior part of the *pituitary gland*. They in turn are controlled by a small structure close by at the base of the brain — the *hypothalamus* — which mediates environmental, stress and emotional factors.

Now let's look at the sequence of events in the cycle and the underlying hormonal changes. By convention the cycle begins with menstruation, although, in biological thinking, it in fact *ends* with menstruation.

The follicle-stimulating hormone (FSH) is secreted from the pituitary and a number of follicles in the ovary ripen and produce oestrogen. Of these, only one grows to maturity. As the oestrogen increases, it has a number of effects:

- The lining of the uterus (endometrium) regenerates and thickens (proliferative phase).
- The cervix ripens and fertile mucus is produced.
- The lining of the vagina is restored and female body features ('secondary sexual characteristics') are sustained.
- Further production of FSH is stopped.

As the oestrogen peaks, it triggers the pituitary gland to produce a surge in luteinizing hormone (LH): ovulation usually follows within four to sixty-four hours (see Figure 18).

The other effect of LH is to secure the formation of the corpus luteum — the yellow body formed after the egg is released. The corpus luteum secretes a small amount of oestrogen, and larger

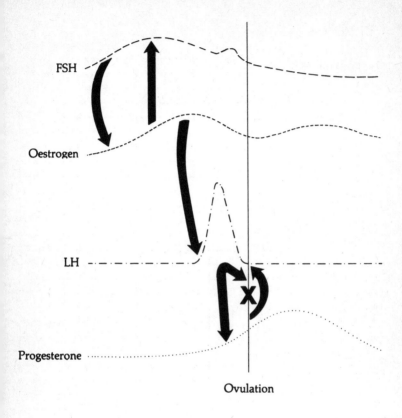

FSH

Oestrogen

LH

Progesterone

Ovulation

Figure 18.   The sequence of hormone changes.

amounts of progesterone, which prepares the way for a possible pregnancy by:

- Causing a rise in body temperature.
- Inhibiting the anterior pituitary and therefore the ripening and release of any further eggs.
- Softening the thickened endometrium (secretory phase).
- Closing off the cervix and thickening the mucus.

As the progesterone and oestrogen fall to low levels, the temperature drops, the endometrium is shed and a new cycle begins.

Figure 19.   A blank chart for your own use.

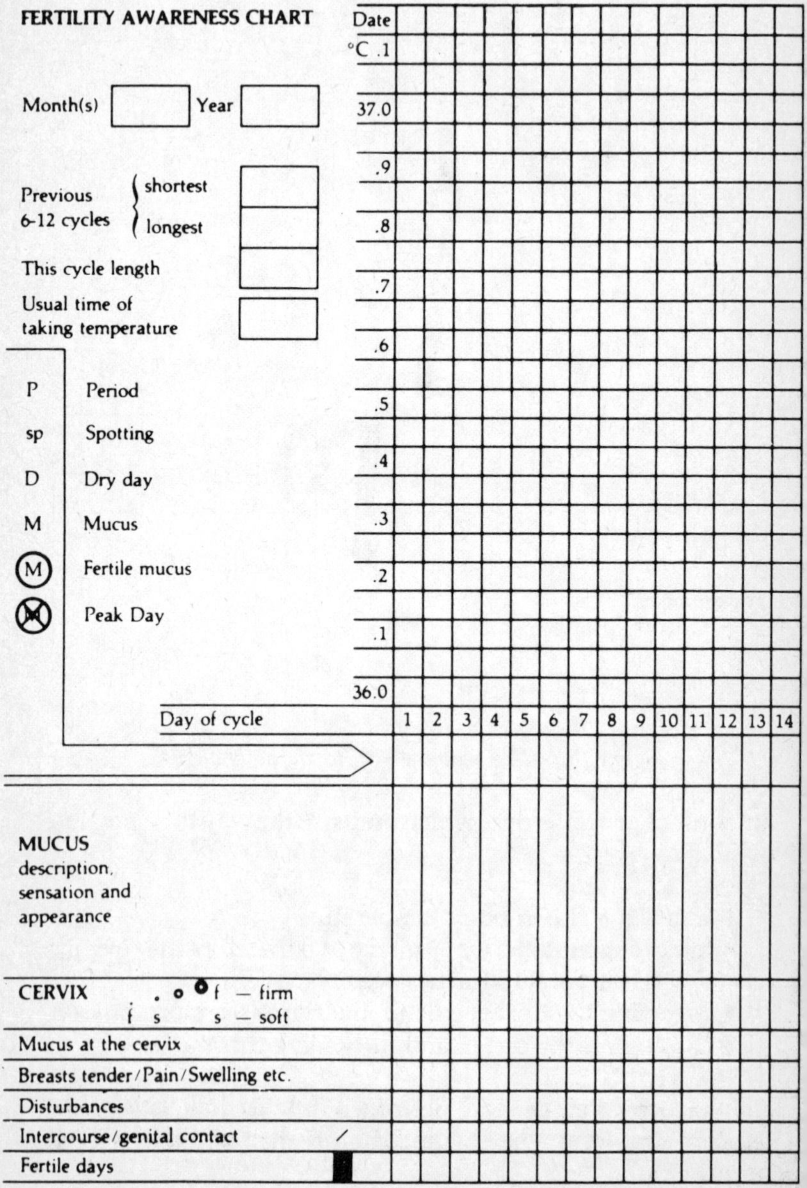

FERTILITY AWARENESS CHART

Month(s) [   ]   Year [   ]

Previous 6-12 cycles { shortest [   ]   longest [   ]

This cycle length [   ]

Usual time of taking temperature [   ]

P	Period
sp	Spotting
D	Dry day
M	Mucus
(M)	Fertile mucus
(M)	Peak Day

Date | °C .1 | 37.0 | .9 | .8 | .7 | .6 | .5 | .4 | .3 | .2 | .1 | 36.0

Day of cycle: 1 2 3 4 5 6 7 8 9 10 11 12 13 14

MUCUS
description,
sensation and
appearance

CERVIX   f — firm   s — soft

Mucus at the cervix

Breasts tender/Pain/Swelling etc.

Disturbances

Intercourse/genital contact

Fertile days

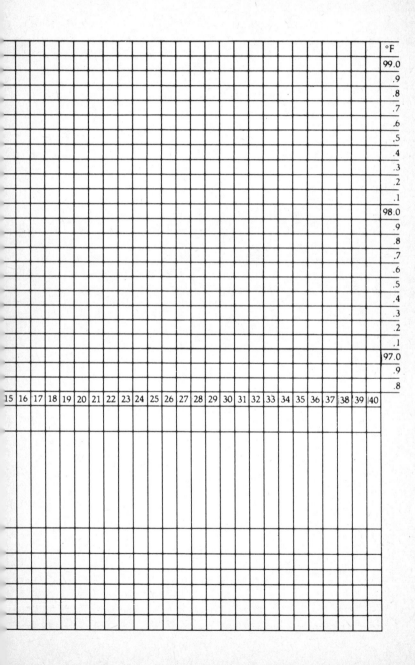

Further Reading

Natural Family Planning

Dr Elizabeth Clubb and Jane Knight, *Fertility: A Comprehensive Guide to Natural Family Planning* (David and Charles, 1987).

Dr Evelyn Billings and Ann Westmore, *The Billings Method* (Penguin, 1982).

Dr Anna Flynn and Melissa Brooks, *A Manual of Natural Family Planning* (Allen and Unwin, 1984).

John and Sheila Kippley, *The Art of Natural Family Planning* (The Couple to Couple League, 1979).

Dr Josef Roetzer, *Some Fine Points of the Symptothermal Method of NFP, 1 and 2* (Human Life Foundation, St Johns University, Collegeville, Mn 56321, U.S.A., 1977-8).

Mary Shivanandan, *Natural Sex* (Hamlyn, 1979).

Reviews of the Main Research on NFP

Periodic Abstinence for Family Planning (International Planned Parenthood Federation Medical Publications, 1983).

Hanna Klaus, Natural Family Planning: a Review (*Obstetrical and Gynaecological Survey 37*, 2, 1982).

Periodic Abstinence: How Well do the New Approaches Work? (*Population Reports Series 1*, 3, 1981).

Paul Thyma, *History of the Biological Control of Human Fertility* (Married Life Information, 1 Manor Drive, Oak Ridge, N.J., U.S.A., 1982).

Contraception

Penny Kane, *The Which? Guide to Birth Control* (Consumers Association, 1983).

John Guillebaud, *Contraception: Your Questions Answered*, (Pitman, 1985).

B. and G. Seaman, *Women and the Crisis in Sex Hormones* (Rawson Associates, New York, 1977).

Female Cycles

Penelope Shuttle and Peter Redgrove, *The Wise Wound: Menstruation and Everywoman* (Gollancz, 1978).

Paula Weideger, *Female Cycles* (The Women's Press, 1975).

The Menopause

Rosetta Reitz, *Menopause: a Positive Approach* (Allen and Unwin, 1977).

Difficulty Conceiving

Dr Andrew Stanway, *Why Us?* (Granada, 1980).

Naomi Pfeffer and Anne Woollet, *The Experience of Infertility* (Virago, 1983).

General Background Reading

Fact Sheets (Family Planning Information Service, 27/35 Mortimer Street, London W1).

Angela Phillips and Jill Rakusen, *Our Bodies Ourselves* (British edition of the Boston Women's Health Collective title, Penguin, 1987).

Thomas Szasz, *Sex: Facts, Frauds and Follies* (Basil Blackwell, Oxford, 1980).

Brian Inglis and Ruth West, *The Alternative Health Guide* (Michael Joseph, 1983).

Useful Addresses

Birmingham NFP Centre, Queen Elizabeth Medical Centre, Birmingham B15 2TG.

NFP Service, Catholic Marriage Advisory Council, 15 Lansdowne Road, London W11 3AJ. (For your local CMAC, refer to the phone book.)

Fertility Awareness Methods Teachers, trained by **Katia and Jonathan Drake,** 12 Priestley House, Athlone Street, London NW5 4LP.

The Family Planning Information Service, 27/35 Mortimer Street, London W1N 7RJ.

Foresight (The Association for the Promotion of Preconceptual Care), The Old Vicarage, Church Lane, Witley, Godalming, Surrey GU8 5PN.

The Birth Centre, 16 Simpson Street, London SW11.

The National Childbirth Trust, 9 Queensborough Terrace, London W2 3TB.

La Leche League (breastfeeding counsellors), Box 3424, London WC1 6XX.

Note: All these organizations would appreciate a stamped addressed envelope with any enquiry!

Rite Time Ltd, 10 Manor Rd, Chatham, Kent ME4 6AL.

Boots Celltech Diagnostics, 240 Bath Rd, Slough, Berkshire, SL1 4ET.

Index

Page numbers in *italics* refer to figures